SHELMAR PUBLICATIONS
BOX 18  1122 WILLARD AVE.
GENOA, NE 68640
1 800 664-1077

# How to Find Your Perfect Job in Nursing

### by Shelly Burke, RN, BSN,
### and Martha Whited, RN, ADN

Library of Congress
Catalog Card No. 96-93078


ISBN 1-57579-052-1

Printed in United States of America

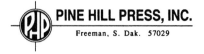 **PINE HILL PRESS, INC.**
Freeman, S. Dak. 57029

# Dedication

To Mom and Dad, Michael, Ashley, and Whitney

To Mom and Dad, Tim, Cody, and Morgan

This book is dedicated to our families—our parents who taught us how to love, and our husbands and children, who taught us how to take care of others.

Nov. 15, 1996

# Acknowledgements

Many thanks to the following people who provided us with; information, contributions, suggestions, listening ears, support, and encouragement. Without your help we could not have fulfilled our dream of writing *How to Find Your Perfect Job in Nursing.*

Anne Burke, Anita Kaspar, Jean Beyer, Rose Waddell, Carol Maddix, Jim Parker, Dee Dee Logue, Teressa Williams, Bev Bergum, Lee Jenkins, Kathy Engel, Terry Lasseter, Katherine Smith, Terry Lahnstein, Donna Nickel, Linda Edelman, Capt. Neva Westhoff, Maj. Carol Amadeo.

Lori Sindelar, Laura Hardy, Alice Plettner, Shelly Boss, Treva Jacobsen, Susan Mark, Pam Nicholls, Debbie Trammell, Lynn Lamp, Barbara Hilb, Cathy Holder, Kate Jones, Kathy Buntin, Lois Keas, Flora Bolin, Frieda Forsman, Mary Dean, Annette Davis, Gayle Hart, Cyndi Rogers, Paulette Hendricks, Tamra Boettcher, Dana Crispin.

Cinda Sorenson, Cyndi Green, Dennis Kennedy, Mary Jo Veskrna, Pat Green, Kathy Hellbusch, Nancy Praeuner, Pam Reese, Chris Vandenberg, Ron Orent, Geri Hansen, Theresa Pinson, Linda Lukesh.

Diane Woods, Phyllis Wingo, Wade and Donna Edwards, Oprah Winfrey, Kent Frenzen, Jim Scow of Scow, Kuhlman, Rief, and Kruse, Lt. Amy Price.

Tom and Dorothy Dutton, Anna Kamp, Michael and Whitney Whited and Ashley Latimer, Terry and Amy Grigsby, Kevin, Cathy and Zachary Dutton and Brad Philpott, Sam and Jennifer Totten.

Pastor and Mrs. Allen Geil, Tim, Cody, and Morgan Burke, Deb Ritter, Becky Geil, Mr. and Mrs. Edward Geil, Mr. and Mrs. Walter Christian, John Christian.

Special thanks to Anne Burke and Ashley Latimer for countless hours of babysitting!

# Table of Contents

## SECTION TWO: WHERE DO I BELONG?
## WHAT ARE MY OPTIONS?
## CHOOSING THE AREA FOR YOUR PERFECT JOB

## SECTION THREE: LANDING YOUR PERFECT JOB

# Preface

To nurses everywhere, who care for patients, doctors,

families, other nurses—everyone but themselves.

## SECTION ONE

# What *Is* Your Perfect Job?
# Defining Your Perfect Job

# RX: Read This Book!

So you've decided to become a nurse. Or maybe you've made it through Anatomy and Physiology, learned to write Care Plans, and given the dreaded first shot, and now all that stands between you and your first real patient is "Boards." Or perhaps you've been a nurse for awhile, but as of yet, have not been able to figure out exactly where in nursing you belong—or have even determined your options!

The career of nursing offers such a wide range of diverse options that it is often hard to know exactly what your Perfect Job is. This is, however, one of the most desirable aspects of the nursing field, for with so many options available, you will never have to feel limited! Knowing what's perfect for *you* at any given time in your life and career, though, is a completely different matter.

The process of finding your Perfect Job in nursing is much more than reading the want ads, writing your resume, filling out an application, and attending an interview. Before you consider those traditional, and yes, important approaches, you must evaluate your personal, family, and professional needs. You must also identify your strengths and weaknesses, likes and dislikes—to name just a few—to determine the specifications of your Perfect Job.

Often the process of elimination alone will help you avoid the misery of choosing an area of nursing that is inherently wrong for you. By eliminating those areas, and narrowing the areas in which you think you may enjoy working, you have already increased your chances of finding an area in which you will thrive. The area or areas that are optimal for *your* consideration will be referred to as your Target Area(s).

It is important to work through this book beginning with Section One, as each section builds on the work you will have completed in the previous section.

In Section One, we will help you determine your Target Areas. Whether you are job hunting for the first time or have been a nurse for some time, taking the time to define your basic needs and goals is absolutely essential in defining your Perfect Job. A variety of tools—quizzes, worksheets, questions to think about, and detailed information to read, will help you hone in on your Target Area(s). We have strived to present these tools in an easy-to-use and informative way. We will guide you through job decisions that *you* need to make; such as, will you work in a direct or indirect patient care area, part-time or full-time, as a floor nurse or on a specialty unit?

We will provide you with basic facts: pros, cons, and other pertinent information that will help you determine the answers to these questions (and more) . . . As you work through Section One, you will record your answers on the "My Perfect Job" worksheet. After you have completed Section One, this worksheet will give you a clear view of the parameters of your Perfect Job—your "must have" aspects, and other features on which you may be willing to compromise. If this sounds overwhelming, don't worry—at the end of the section we illustrate how several nurses completed this process and determined the requirements for their Perfect Job.

Section Two contains a comprehensive listing of job opportunities for nurses. By learning about these areas— what the job involves, the pros and cons of each different area of expertise, and many other factors to consider—you will be able to further narrow your Target Area.

After working through Sections One and Two, you will have a *clear* picture of the aspects your Perfect Job will include. Section Three will help you find—and get—that job!

In Section Three, we have included tips on how to create not just a standard resume, but a unique and effective resume! We have provided you with information and suggestions to make the interview work for you. Most importantly, we have provided you with a way to compare job offers and determine which one is your Perfect Job. We call this the "Your Perfect Job Comparison Worksheet" and you will find it an invaluable tool in mapping your future success.

Finding your Perfect Job in Nursing may seem like an overwhelming challenge, but relax! Take a deep breath, grab a pencil and just consider this a field trip—to your frontal lobe! The time you spend working through this book will pay off with a tremendous reward—your next job will be Your Perfect Job in Nursing!

# How to Use This Section

Section one is designed to help you define your Target Area—specifications of your Perfect Job. First we will help you define your personal, family, and career needs and goals. Don't be tempted to rush through this section—take your time! Working within your needs and goals is the basis of your Perfect Job. It may take several hours, or even several days to define these goals; and you will need to re-evaluate your needs and goals periodically as they may drastically change over time!

If you find you need a break from working on your needs and goals, skip ahead and look at some of the information presented in the second half of Section One. Here you will determine more guidelines for your Perfect Job. Do you want to work full-time or part-time? In a small or large facility? Which shift? We have presented some of the information in the form of pros and cons, reasons the area may or may *not* be for you, and other pertinent information to consider. Other information is presented in quiz form—but don't worry—unlike microbiology or patient teaching there are no wrong answers, only answers that are right for *you!*

At the end of each chapter, there is a space for "Personal notes/comments" to jot down any additional factors that will influence your decision regarding the issue being discussed.

After you've finished each quiz or worksheet, remember to transfer your answer to the "My Perfect Job" worksheet on page 173.

# Soul Searching:
# Assessing Your Personal, Family, and Professional Needs and Goals

*"To be a good care giver, one must first take care of herself. If a nurse does not keep her life in balance, she "burns out" and therefore is not able to be effective with her cares."* Bev Bergum, R.N.

Your Perfect Job must fit in with your personal, family, and professional needs and goals. By taking a hard look at these areas in your life, and through filling out the worksheets in this chapter, you will determine the priority needs and goals in these areas of your life. You will then have a better understanding of your Perfect Job parameters. The following questions will help to stimulate your thought processes. The quizzes and worksheets will further help you define your needs and goals (and yes, you do have them!) This is the heart of your Perfect Job. Soul-searching to determine needs and goals is a private and individualized journey. The more thought you put into this area of the book, the more harmonious your life will become. So find a quiet place, clear your mind—and don't forget to bring your pencil.

# Determining Personal Needs And Goals:
## What Do *I* Want Out Of Life?

*"Be honest with yourself first—don't try to be something you're not."* Anita Kaspar, L.P.N

At times it may seem as if your personal needs and goals are forgotten or non-existent when compared to the many needs of your family and job. Sound familiar? If so, are you happy? The U.S. Constitution guarantees every U.S. citizen the right to the pursuit of happiness; therefore, it is not only constitutional to pursue happiness—it's un-American not to!

It is necessary to be fulfilled *personally* before you can successfully meet the needs of others. To begin your personal assessment, be decadent! Think only of yourself as you consider and answer the statements below.

* List three personal needs. These are your basic personality needs, and the ability to have these needs met is directly related to how you feel about yourself and the other areas of your life. (Examples: need time alone every day, need to spend time with family)

* List three short-term goals you hope to accomplish within the next six months (remember—not related to family or nursing) (Examples: attend aerobics class three times every week; pay off credit card bill)

* List three long-term goals you hope to accomplish within the next five years (Examples: buy a new car; learn how to refinish furniture)

* List three things about yourself you would like to improve (Examples: lose 10 pounds; gain confidence in social situations)

* List the three most important activities/events you attend (may include family activities) (Examples: Thanksgiving family reunion, church activities)

* List five personality traits (Examples: need time to myself; enjoy being with children; work well under pressure)

* * * * * * * * * * * * * * * * * * * *

By thinking about and writing down these personal needs, goals, and characteristics, you will have a clearer picture of what makes you happy. Now that you have done this, congratulate yourself—you have identified *your* needs and goals. As you consider different jobs, think about how each job will fit within your personal needs and goals.

# Identifying Family Needs And Goals:
## What Do *They* Need And Want?

If you have a partner, spouse, and/or children, the parameters for your Perfect Job may be more narrow. If your children are young, your job may have to fit around available day care. If your children are older, your Perfect Job may need to allow you to attend activities in which your children are involved.

Regardless of the presence of a spouse, and/or ages of your children, you need to consider the self-sufficiency of your family. If family members are willing and able to help with cooking, cleaning, and shopping, your search for the Perfect Job may be easier, as you can be more flexible about the number of hours, and which hours, you spend at work. If family members are unwilling or unable to help out, you may need to work fewer hours so that you can manage those unending household tasks.

If nearby relatives are willing to assist with child care and perhaps errands or housework, you won't need to be so concerned about regular day-care providers calling in sick, or dust bunnies overtaking your house. Have an honest discussion with your relatives, though, before you count on them to help; just because they live nearby does not guarantee they will be willing to help.

To assess family needs and goals:

* List three *family* needs that must be met for your family to remain stable (Examples: eat meals together three or four times every week to discuss family issues; attend church activities)

* List three short-term family goals you would like to achieve within the next six months (Example: remodel the family room; construct a volleyball court in the back yard)

*   List three long-term family goals you would like to reach in the next five years (Examples: family trip to Disneyland; save money for son who starts college in three years)

*   List several of the most important activities you do as a family (Examples: attend soccer games and band concerts; two-week camp in the summer)

*   When do most of these activities take place? During the day? Evening? During the week? Mostly on weekends? Are they seasonal, or do they occur throughout the year?

* * * * * * * * * * * * * * * * * * * *

Your family may participate in just a few, seasonal activities (sports, camp). If so, you may be able to get time off to attend these events by requesting it or trading shifts with another nurse. However, if your family takes part in many activities throughout the year, you may need to choose a shift that will allow you to attend the majority of those activities (for example, working the day or night shift so you can attend evening activities).

A slight modification in your work schedule can make a *big* difference. While twelve-hour shifts mean an extended time away from home, more days and evenings are free for family activities. Working just one or two shifts a week less may make a significant difference, as may working only weekends, leaving weekdays free for attending activities.

Remember, if your family is unhappy because you cannot attend important events—or you are so stressed in trying to balance work, family, and home—you will not be happy with your job.

* * * * * * * * * * * * * * * * * * * *

9

# Defining Professional Needs And Goals:
# What Do *I* Want Out Of Nursing?

A career in nursing offers endless job options. You may want to gain experience in many different areas, or work for a specialty certification. Your goal may be to attain a Charge Nurse position, or you may desire to work in a management position. Perhaps you want to further your education and earn an advanced degree. In nursing, you can reach one, or all, of these goals!

Your career can go in any direction. However, if you do *not* choose a direction, you may liken yourself to a boat afloat without an anchor. Begin by defining your career needs and goals and listing the steps for reaching these goals. Don't worry about making a wrong decision—your goals can and may change at any time over the course of your career. All you have to lose by not defining your career goals is finding that special area in which you can grow professionally and makes you feel unequivocally good about your career.

To assess career needs and goals:

*   List three career needs. If you are a new graduate, or haven't worked in the field of nursing for some time, think back on clinical or other nursing experiences to determine career needs (Example: relatively low-stress job; supportive manager; opportunity for learning)

*   List three short-term career goals you hope to accomplish within the next six months (Examples: become comfortable with hospital routine; learn to administer chemotherapy; attend ACLS classes)

*   Pick the most important goal(s) you listed and map out the steps you will take to attain those goal(s)

*   List three to five long-term goals you hope to achieve within the next five years (Examples: become certified as a CCRN—Critical Care Registered Nurse; begin school towards a Masters Degree)

*   Select your two most important goals (make sure they are compatible!) and map out the steps you will take to attain these goals. List *every* step you will have to take (for example, attaining an advanced degree involves; determining classes you need to take; determining colleges offering the class, etc.)

\* \* \* \* \* \* \* \* \* \* \* \* \* \* \* \* \* \* \* \*

Before committing yourself to a specific goal, consider what is actually involved in reaching that goal. Perhaps getting a specialty certification requires having an advanced degree; getting an advanced degree may mean traveling long distances to classes, and so on. After considering the time, cost, and effort involved, you may choose to cut down on work hours, allowing you the time to attend classes. Or you may decide to delay the goal for some time, or even choose a different, more realistic goal, to work toward.

\* \* \* \* \* \* \* \* \* \* \* \* \* \* \* \* \* \* \* \*

# Your Vision—Pulling It All Together

Now, how will these worksheets help you find your Perfect Job? We have guided you in defining your personal, family, and career needs and goals; now you have to decide how *you* will use your answers!

What are your top priorities and most important goals, at this time? (remember, your goals and priorities will change over time). If your greatest priorities are related to financial needs or goals, you will probably choose to accept a high paying job, no matter what shift or area it is in. If your primary goals are family oriented, you will search for and accept a job which will allow you to be with your family as much as possible, regardless of pay or area. If your priority is to advance your career, you will choose a job that will help meet this goal, regardless of pay or shift.

To complicate matters, most of us are working on several goals at one time, and they may be difficult to prioritize.

Reading through the following situations will help you see your goals and priorities more clearly.

* Lisa, 24, is married and has no children. She and her husband would like to buy a house within the next five years (long-term family goal) and begin their own family within a year (long-term family goal). Lisa would like to finish paying off her school loan within the next six months (short-term personal goal) and take several business classes through the local college next semester (short-term personal goal).

    Lisa just graduated from nursing school and would like a job in any area in which she can perfect her basic skills of medication administration, assessment, IV skills, etc.

    Lisa decides that her most important goals are financial. She decides to look for a high-paying job, regardless of shift or area of nursing. Because her greatest priority is earning and saving money, she will work her class schedule around her work schedule.

* Sharon, 43, is married and has three children; 13, 16, and 18 years old. Her children are involved in many school activities, and her 18 year-old will graduate from high-school in the spring. Sharon worked at a small hospital, but her sched-

ule is erratic and the pay is low, compared to that of larger facilities.

Sharon's main priority is to spend time with her family (long-term family goal), and she would like to earn more money to help her son with college expenses (short-term family and personal goal). Sharon would also like to have more time to work on craft projects (personal goal) and although she has worked in many areas of nursing, would like to try a critical care area (short-term career goal).

Sharon decides to look for a job with twelve-hour shifts, in critical care. Her older children are self-sufficient and willing to help with housework, and by working twelve-hour shifts Sharon will only have to work three days a week, leaving ample time for family activities. As an added bonus, Sharon will be working towards two goals—financial and career—by getting a job in a higher paying area.

* Joy, 33, is the single mother of children ages two, five, and six. She receives child-support but needs to work about 30 hours a week to make ends meet. She is very active in her local church. Joy has been a nurse for 11 years, working in the local nursing home. However, twelve-hour shifts were recently instituted, and Joy cannot find child care for that extended period of time.

Joy's main priorities are finding a Monday through Friday job with traditional day hours (long-term family need and goal) for ease of finding child care, and so they can continue to participate in church activities.

Joy decides to focus her search on doctor's offices and clinics, as they are open the hours she prefers to work. She also inquires at local nursing homes, as many "paperwork" jobs require only day hours.

\* \* \* \* \* \* \* \* \* \* \* \* \* \* \* \* \* \* \* \*

See, that wasn't so difficult! Now it's *your* turn to pull it all together.

* List your greatest personal need:

*   List your greatest personal goal:



*   List your greatest family need:



*   List your greatest family goal:



*   List your greatest career need:



*   List your greatest career goal:




How do you see your Perfect Job fitting within these priority needs and goals?



* * * * * * * * * * * * * * * * * * *

Congratulations! You have completed the most important part of finding your Perfect Job. Needs and goals can—and will—change, and certain needs and goals will take precedence at different times in your life.

The following chapters provide quizzes, worksheets, and more information to help you further define your Perfect Job. However, your personal, family, and career priorities will remain the corner-stone of your search.

* * * * * * * * * * * * * * * * * * *

# Utilizing The Hidden Advantages: Benefitting From Benefits

Benefits are services or additional pay available to employees either at a reduced rate or free. Benefits are an often overlooked, but very important, part of an employment package. Rather than asking about benefits after you accept a job, request a list of benefits when a job offer has been extended, so that you may consider them as an *integral part* of your job offer, and not as an afterthought.

Benefits that may be offered include: (terms are defined in the Glossary)

\_\_\_Health Insurance

\_\_\_Life Insurance

\_\_\_Disability/Dismemberment Insurance

\_\_\_Dental Insurance

\_\_\_Vision Plan

\_\_\_Maternity/Paternity Leave

\_\_\_On-Site Child-Care or Child-Care Assistance

\_\_\_Holidays

\_\_\_Vacation Days

\_\_\_Sick Days

\_\_\_Personal Time Off (PTO)

\_\_\_Shift Differential

\_\_\_Charge Nurse Differential

\_\_\_Differential for nurses with advanced degrees

\_\_\_"On Call" pay

\_\_\_Reduced rates for hospital services

\_\_\_Credit Union

\_\_\_Recruitment Bonus

\_\_\_Relocation Assistance

___Housing Assistance

___Uniform Allowance

___Pension Plan

___Flexible Scheduling/Job Sharing

___Orientation, Refresher Courses, Internship, Preceptorship

___Career Ladder

___Education Assistance

___Personal improvement classes; stop-smoking, weight loss, stress management, etc.

___Reduced fees at area gym facilities or local classes

___Discounted or free meals in the facility cafeteria

___Free parking

Benefits vary widely from facility to facility. Part-time employees usually receive fewer benefits than full-time employees. Larger facilities usually offer a wider range of benefits; however, smaller facilities may offer recruitment bonuses and more flexible work hours. Hospitals usually have better benefits than out-of-hospital facilities such as privately owned Home Health agencies.

If you have questions about what benefits are offered and how they work, make an appointment to speak with the Personnel Director or Human Resource Person, who will answer any questions you may have. Until you have a clear understanding of *all* benefits, you cannot make an informed decision about a job offer.

Never consider hourly wage or salary alone! A good benefit package can more than make up for a lower wage, while a job that pays a higher wage may offer fewer benefits.

Carefully consider the benefits which are a priority to you. Health insurance is a priority to many people, whereas on-site child-care may be a higher priority to a mother whose husband's employer provides health insurance.

Do not consider just the benefits that you will use immediately. If you plan to have a family someday, ask about maternity and paternity leave and on-site child-care. If you would like to continue your education, check into the possibility of education assistance.

* * * * *

Lynn was impressed with the insurance package a certain hospital offered. She accepted a job at this hospital, in large part, due to these benefits. Unfortunately, she didn't do her homework thoroughly. After she started her new job and cancelled her personal insurance policy, she realized that she didn't qualify for insurance with her new employer until she had been working for three months. She faced buying her own insurance for that amount of time, or going without.

Another nurse, Susan, had been employed elsewhere for about five months when her Perfect Job opportunity opened up in her home town. Luckily, before she gave her two-week notice, Susan spoke with the Personnel Director. She found that vacation and sick hours could only be converted to cash after working 1,040 hours at the facility. By working one additional week, along with the traditional two-week notice, Susan reached this magical number. It was like winning the lottery! She converted her sick and vacation hours to cold, hard cash, and promptly purchased a new washing machine, dryer, and dishwasher for her new home. What a bonus, just for knowing to ask the right questions.

* * * * *

So always be aware that benefits of any kind are only as good as is your understanding of them. Without your understanding, you will not be able to make the most of your "hidden advantages."

After considering your personal, family, and career needs and goals, number from one to five (with one being your top priority benefit) the benefits which are of the greatest priority to you. Transfer your priority benefits to the "My Perfect Job" worksheet on page 173 of this book.

* * * * * * * * * * * * * * * * * * * *

Personal notes/comments:

# To Drive Or Not To Drive: Considering Commuting?

Unless you are lucky enough to live within blocks of your Perfect Job, you will need to make a decision regarding commuting—Yes, No, or under what circumstances you would consider commuting—early in your job search.

To drive . . .

If you enjoy driving, have a reliable vehicle, and the extra time spent commuting still allows you to meet your personal and family needs, the decision to commute is easy.

If you live in a rural area in which there is no hospital, long-term care unit, or medical clinic, then commuting will be a necessity. If there *is* a hospital or other health-care facility, job openings may be limited, also making commuting a necessity. Even in a larger city, commuting may be necessary due to the requirements of the jobs available, or to meet personal, family, or career needs or goals.

If you are willing to commute, you need to determine how far, geographically, you are willing to commute. Remember, it's unrealistic to commute four hours each way to an eight-hour a day job!

Don't rule out a great job in a far-off facility just because it involves a commute. Julie found her Perfect Job in a children's psychiatric hospital 45 miles from her home. She expressed her interest in the job and her reservations about driving an extra hour to and from the job five days a week. The interviewer told her about the "weekend plan" the facility offered; an employee could commit to working two, twelve-hour shifts *every* weekend. For working 24 hours, the employee was paid for 36 hours of work and received full-time benefits. Julie gladly accepted the job. The long commute was worth it, as Julie could attend school and family activities during the week—her main reason for *not* wanting to commute (because she would miss many activities) had been resolved!

. . . or not to drive . . .

Perhaps you will find it easy to decide *against* commuting—you don't like to drive, or don't want to spend extra time driving.

If your car is unreliable, or you live in a climate where adverse weather conditions are a regular occurrence (and you don't like to drive in them) and nursing opportunities close to home are comparable to jobs farther away, you may decide you definitely do *not* want to commute. Then, you can focus your job search on health care facilities close to home.

. . . there is a question!

It is likely, though, that many factors will be a part of your decision whether or not to commute. A "dream job" in a specialty hospital may be well worth a substantial drive. Commuting to a larger city may be advantageous as hospitals in a larger city may offer higher wages or better benefits that will more than outweigh the money spent for gas, wear and tear on your car, and other expenses associated with commuting.

If you would consider commuting, decide under what circumstances you would commute; would it depend on pay, the specific job, working in a particular hospital, or working certain hours? You must decide how commuting fits in with your list of priorities.

So, to drive or not to drive, that is the question—and only *you* have the answer.

* * * * *

The following questions will help you further clarify your decision to commute—or not, and the conditions under which you would consider commuting.

### Personal

Do you enjoy driving?

Do you consider "drive time" an opportunity to prepare for and unwind from work, or do you look at it as taking time away from personal and family activities?

How far are you willing to commute?

Miles_____
     *   Using a protractor and pencil, draw a circle on a map en-
        compassing this area. Your Perfect Job is waiting in a
        health-care facility in this circle!

Minutes_____


Would you rather drive within a city or on the interstate or other roads outside of the city? Does it matter to you?


### Driving

Is your car comfortable, and easy to drive?


Is your car reliable?


How many miles does your car have? Do you mind putting more miles on your car?


For each job you are considering, figure how many miles you will be driving in a week, month, year. Are you willing to put these extra miles on your car?


What is the condition of the roads on which you will drive? Are they well maintained? Do they need work? If they are scheduled for repair, this may mean detours and/or delays (adding more time and miles to your commute).

Will you be driving in snow, rain, or other adverse weather conditions? Are you comfortable driving in these adverse conditions?

## Money

Is your pay sufficient to cover the extra costs of commuting—gas, car maintenance, longer hours of child care?

*OR* Are the career opportunities you are offered enough to make up for the extra costs of commuting?

## Career

Can you reach your career goals easier/faster by commuting?

* * * * * * * * * * * * * * * * * * * *

Personal notes/comments:

# CONCERNING COMMUTING

Please circle the appropriate statement below:

I am *not* willing to commute

* * *

I am willing to commute

* * *

I am willing to commute under the following conditions

I will commute _____ miles to my Perfect Job

I will commute _____ minutes/hours to my Perfect Job

Other conditions:

Please transfer the answer(s) to the "My Perfect Job" worksheet on page 173 of this book.

# Narrowing Your Target Area: Scoping Out Your Options

## How Much Should You Work?

One of the first decisions to make during your quest for the Perfect Job is whether you want (or need) to work part-time or full-time. This decision, as well as the others you will be making in this section, will depend on your personal, family, and professional needs and goals. This chapter will present pros and cons of working part-time vs. full-time.

### PART-TIME

Depending on facility policy, you are usually considered a part-time employee if you work less than 32 hours per week; check facility policy.

Pros:
* don't get burned out as easily
* not as physically or mentally demanding
* you may get paid more per hour in lieu of receiving benefits
* working part-time allows you to earn money and retain nursing skills while having more time for family or other activities
* depending on the number of hours you work every week you may work another part-time or even full-time job
* you may be required to work fewer weekends and holidays than a person working full-time
* working part-time allows you to "try out" a job before committing to it full-time

Cons:
* you may be assigned to uncooperative or difficult patients from whom regular staff members need a break
* may receive few or no benefits
* less continuity with patients, staff members, and any facility/floor/unit issues

Part-time work may be for you if:
* you have many family or other commitments outside of work
* you physically cannot work full-time
* you hold another full-time or part-time job

Part-time work may *not* be for you if:
* you need benefits such as health insurance or social security

Other information to consider:
Management positions usually require full-time employment and working part-time is not an option.

A part-time employee may have the opportunity to work more hours if the area is short-staffed. Part-time options may be very flexible; some facilities offer the option to work weekends only, or a certain number of weekends a month. If a similar arrangement would benefit you, ask your interviewer about these options.

* * * * * * * * * * * * * * * * * * * *

Personal notes/comments:

## FULL-TIME

An employee working 32 hours per week or more is usually considered full-time; again, check facility policy.

Pros:
* full-time wages and benefits
* continuity with patients, staff, and floor/unit/facility issues

Cons:
* less time for family and other commitments
* you will be required to work weekends and holidays (check facility policy)
* working full-time is more physically and mentally demanding than working part-time

24

This chapter lists the general hours of each shift, (facility policy may vary) pros and cons of each shift, why the shift may or may not be for you, and other factors to consider. Take time to consider the information presented. If you accept a job where the hours don't accommodate your lifestyle, you are sure to be stressed out—physically and mentally! Neither you, your employer, your co-workers, or your patients will benefit from this.

Please keep in mind that these are only guidelines; occasionally a day shift may be as quiet as a night shift and a night shift may include three emergency admissions and/or surgeries!

## DAY SHIFT

Hours: 6 AM-2 PM; 7 AM-3 PM; 8 AM-4 PM

Pros:
* working these hours leaves evenings free for family or other activities
* child care is readily available during these hours
* many opportunities to use and perfect technical skills—IV's, NG's, dressing changes, etc.
* support staff—doctors, respiratory therapists, other nurses, and so on, are readily available if you have questions or problems

Cons:
* the shift is very busy; daily hygiene and linen changes are done, two meals are served, the majority of tests, surgeries, admissions, and dismissals are done during this shift
* the work is physically demanding—you may be on your feet most of the day
* pay is the lowest of all shifts
* doctors, staff from different departments, and administrative staff are in the building and have the potential to disrupt your day

The day shift may be for you if:
* you like to get up early
* you are a new grad or new to a particular clinical area; you will get ample opportunity to perfect your technical skills and observe and assist with procedures

* you like the fast pace
* you have good prioritizing and organizational skills, or want to work on improving these skills

The day shift may *not* be for you if:
* you do not like to get up early
* you like a more relaxed pace of work
* it is difficult for you to keep up physically with a tremendous work load

Other factors to consider:
* Regardless of the area and shift you plan to eventually go to, working the day shift gives you the opportunity to perfect technical skills in the shortest amount of time, and numerically has the greatest availability of experienced nurses to assist and answer questions.

* * * * * * * * * * * * * * * * * * * *

Personal notes/comments:

## EVENING SHIFT

Hours: 2 PM-10 PM; 3 PM-11 PM; 4 PM-12 AM

Pros:
* you don't have to get up early in the morning (very important if you like to stay out late at night!)
* the pace is slower; you serve one meal and assist the patients with PM cares and settling in for the night
* fewer tests are done during the evening shift; you will usually not have to coordinate transfers to various testing departments but will have an occasional emergency transfer
* with a more relaxed pace, you have more opportunity to interact with your patients
* a shift differential is usually paid for working the evening shift

Cons:
*   you may not be able to attend family or social activities that take place in the evening
*   may have a lot of "fresh" post-op patients, or evening admissions from the ER, who will require frequent vital sign checks and close monitoring
*   the evening shift is often the most difficult shift to staff, which means you will work "short" most often on this shift

The evening shift may be for you if:
*   you do not like to get up early
*   you like to go out late at night after work
*   you like a fair amount of action and patient contact but not the intense activity of days
*   you enjoy interacting with patients and family members; the majority of visitors visit in the evening

The evening shift may *not* be for you if:
*   you have an active social life or family life or attend school in the evening
*   you have small children; it is difficult to find care for children during evening hours

Other factors to consider:
*   Doctors, people from other departments, administrators, etc. may not be in the building but are still relatively easy to reach if needed.

* * * * * * * * * * * * * * * * * * * *

Personal notes/comments:

# NIGHT SHIFT

*"Don't be quick to turn down an 11PM-7AM (night) position. You'll learn more on the night shift than any other shift."* Jim Parker, RN

Hours: 10 PM-6 AM; 11 PM-7 AM; 12 AM-8 AM

Pros:
* the night shift usually has a slow, relaxed pace
* fewer interruptions; you have more time to evaluate your patients, chart, and do care plans
* less physical work with patients; nurses try to encourage regular sleep patterns
* there are few, if any, tests, etc. ordered during the night shift
* usually paid the highest differential

Cons:
* emergencies do occur, and there are less support people available to assist
* the night shift may be hard to adjust to—physically and mentally
* doctors and other "on call" ancillary department personnel may be difficult to deal with if you call them during the night

The night shift may be for you if:
* you are comfortable acting independently, with little support staff immediately available
* you can adjust physically and mentally to the night shift (if you are already a "night person" this will not be a problem for you!)
* you have the "people skills" to talk to doctors in the middle of the night
* you are able to adapt your sleep/wake patterns to job and other commitments

The night shift may *not* be for you if:
* you have small children who will be unsupervised if you sleep during the day
* you like the security of back-up staff being immediately available

*   you want to gain experience with technical skills rapidly
*   you find it difficult to sleep during the day

Other factors to consider:
*   If you can establish alternative sleep patterns, the night shift will not limit or severely affect your daily activities. If you are part of a two-parent family and your spouse works during the day and can be home with young children at night, the night shift may be ideal for you as you will spend less money on child care.

\* \* \* \* \* \* \* \* \* \* \* \* \* \* \* \* \* \* \* \*

Personal notes/comments:

## TWELVE-HOUR SHIFTS

Hours: 6 AM-6 PM; 6 PM-6 AM; 7 AM-7 PM; 7 PM-7 AM

Pros:
*   during a twelve-hour shift you have more time to get charting, procedures, and other tasks done
*   fewer days to work (most facilities consider 36 hours/week to be full-time and will offer full-time benefits; some even pay an employee for 40 hours for working three, twelve-hour shifts)
*   usually work only every third weekend and holiday, rather than every other
*   four days off each week!

Cons:
*   your "holidays on" mean twelve hours away from family
*   if you have children, you may have trouble finding child care for twelve hours (plus commuting time)
*   the long hours can be hard physically and mentally; if you have a long commute you may spend 14 hours away from home each day you work

31

* if the days you work are not continuous, you don't have continuity with patients
* if the days you work are continuous, you may find yourself exhausted!

Twelve-hour shifts may be for you if:
* you have no young dependent children, or have reliable child care available for long hours
* you don't mind working long hours and enjoy having more days off

Twelve-hour shifts may *not* be for you if:
* you don't like working such long hours
* you cannot arrange for child care for extended hours

Other factors to consider:
* Please refer to the other shift outlines for the shifts included in the twelve hour shift that you are considering (day/evening or evening/night).

* * * * * * * * * * * * * * * * * * * * *

Personal notes/comments:

## SHORT SHIFTS

Nurses are needed for short shifts during busy times on the floor, or when a floor is short-staffed for just a few hours; between the time an eight-hour shift ends and the next twelve-hour shift begins, for example. Hours may vary according to facility needs; shifts may be four, six, or ten hours long and usually overlap several shifts; 3 PM-7 PM, for example.

Pros:
* good way to earn a little extra money without committing to a full shift of work
* excellent for students who need study time

Cons:
* it may be difficult to get organized if your short shift begins in the middle of a shift
* it is difficult to get everything done during a short shift

Short shifts may be for you if:
* you don't mind coming or leaving in the middle of a shift
* the hours that extra help is needed are convenient for your schedule

Short shifts may *not* be for you if:
* you have a long commute or need child care; the cost and time of driving and/or child care may not be covered by the short hours worked
* you need *significantly* more income

Other information to consider:
* If you are a new grad or new to the clinical area, short shifts are a way to pick up valuable experience.

* * * * * * * * * * * * * * * * * * * * *

Personal notes/comments:

# DETERMINING YOUR "PERFECT SHIFT"

List the most important factors in your personal life, that will help determine your "perfect shift": (Example: childcare, family activities, night school)

List the most important factors, regarding nursing, that will help determine your "perfect shift": (Example: new grad, prefer quiet shift)

* * * * * * * * * * * * * * * * * * *

From the information in the previous pages, which two shifts would fit into your Perfect Job? (circle two)

Day shift        Evening shift        Night shift

Twelve-hour days        Twelve-hour nights

Short shifts

**Transfer this answer to the "My Perfect Job" worksheet on page 174 of this book.

* * * * * * * * * * * * * * * * * * *

# Where Should You Work?

Before you fill out any applications, you need to decide if you would rather work in a small facility, a large facility, or if facility size is even a priority in your search for your Perfect Job.

Your answers to this quiz will help you assess your preference toward working in a small or large facility.

1. Do you feel comfortable drawing blood, doing respiratory treatments, etc.?
   A. yes
   B. no

2. Do you like to work
   A. with a lot of other people
   B. independently

3. Are you comfortable acting independently during emergencies?
   A. yes
   B. no

4. Do you prefer working with
   A. a variety of patient diagnoses and wide age range
   B. one type of patient

5. Do you like to talk frequently with
   A. doctors, nurses, administrators
   B. nurses, people from other departments

6. Would you like to
   A. be asked to serve on one or more committees
   B. volunteer to serve on a committee

7. What is more important to you?
   A. long-term stability in a job
   B. a close, "family like" relationship with all staff members

8. What is more important to you?

35

A. higher wages, competitive benefits, chance for advancement

B. socially knowing everyone in the whole facility and possibly many of the patients

9.  Do you prefer to
    A. work with many specialty doctors
    B. work with a few general practice doctors

10. Do you prefer
    A. referring to an employee's badge to know his or her name
    B. knowing all employees personally

Answering "A" to questions 1, 3, 4, 5, 6, indicates a preference for working in a small facility.

Answering "A" to questions 2, 7, 8, 9, 10, indicates a preference for working in a large facility.

If seven or more of your answers indicate a preference for working in *either* a small or large facility, you will probably be happier working in a facility of that size. If your answers are almost equally divided, you may choose to apply at several facilities, both large and small, and take the job that fits the majority of your other requirements for your Perfect Job.

\* \* \* \* \* \* \* \* \* \* \* \* \* \* \* \* \* \* \* \* \*

According to this quiz I prefer working in a (circle one):

Small facility                    Large facility

No preference toward

Small or Large facility

**Transfer your answer to the "My Perfect Job" worksheet on page 174 of this book.

\* \* \* \* \* \* \* \* \* \* \* \* \* \* \* \* \* \* \* \* \*

Personal notes/comments:

36

# DO YOU PREFER DIRECT OR INDIRECT PATIENT CARE?

A primary decision you will need to make is determining your preference for working in direct or indirect patient care. Examples of direct "hands on" patient care areas include medical/surgical and pediatrics. Indirect patient care is usually a managerial or "paperwork" position like Director of Nursing or Infection Control. The questions in this quiz point out differences in direct and indirect patient care. Your answers indicate the area in which you are more likely to function well and enjoy.

1. Do you prefer
   A. long-term projects
   B. to see the results of your work every day

2. Would you enjoy attending several meetings every week?
   A. yes
   B. no

3. Regarding paperwork, do you prefer doing
   A. precise, daily charting
   B. comprehensive, long-term tracking

4. Do you prefer working
   A. consistent hours
   B. a variety of hours and shifts

5. Do you prefer communicating with
   A. patients, other nurses, doctors
   B. patients families, nurses, doctors, department heads, administrators

6. Would you rather teach
   A. patients and their families
   B. other nurses

7. On a day-to-day basis, would you rather
   A. administer medications, monitor lab results, maintain IV's, do patient teaching
   B. trouble shoot, problem solve, do paperwork, implement new strategies

8.  Have you worked in an area of direct patient care for at least one year?
    A. yes
    B. no

9.  Do you like to
    A. leave your job at work
    B. be consulted regardless of time of day or night

10. Do you enjoy
    A. problem solving and crises
    B. leaving your job at work

If you answered "A" to questions 3, 5, 6, 7, 9, you seem to prefer areas of direct patient care.

If you answered "A" to questions 1, 2, 4, 8, 10, you seem to prefer areas of indirect patient care.

If seven or more of your answers indicate a preference toward *either* direct or indirect patient care, you will probably be happiest choosing a job in the area indicated. If your answers are split almost evenly between direct and indirect patient care, you may choose to interview for jobs in both types of patient care, and take the job that you feel will be the most fulfilling, or the job that fits the majority of your other requirements for your Perfect Job.

\* \* \* \* \* \* \* \* \* \* \* \* \* \* \* \* \* \* \* \*

According to this quiz I prefer (circle one):

Direct patient care                Indirect patient care

No preference towards Direct or
Indirect patient care

\*\*Transfer this answer to the "My Perfect Job" worksheet on page 174 of this book

\* \* \* \* \* \* \* \* \* \* \* \* \* \* \* \* \* \* \* \*

Personal notes/comments:

38

# GENERAL NURSING OR A SPECIALTY AREA?

General nursing is done on a non-specialty floor, usually medical/surgical. In this area (med/surg) you will be exposed to patients with many types of medical problems— blood clots, decubitus ulcers, pneumonia—or preparing for or recovering from, any type of surgery—gallbladder, hysterectomy, etc.

Small hospitals may not have specialty areas (ICU, OB, etc.) and a nurse working in a small hospital will probably be required to care for patients of all ages with any type of problem or illness.

A nurse working in a specialty area will work with patients who primarily have a specific type of problem—heart problems in a cardiac unit, or psychiatric problems on a psychiatric unit, for example. Nurses who work in a specialty area will develop specialized skills required for that area.

A new graduate may choose to work in a general nursing area so s/he has the opportunity to become experienced at basic nursing skills, be exposed to a variety of procedures, and learn how to deal with difficult situations. Basic nursing allows the nurse to determine, to some extent, with which types of patients s/he enjoys working.

A new graduate, or nurse with little experience, may choose general nursing to gain experience and later choose a specialty area. A nurse with some experience may choose to try a specialty area based upon the skills which s/he enjoys using and the type of patients s/he prefers.

## GENERAL NURSING

Pros:
* greatest diversity of patient care, procedures and skills used

Cons:
* need to learn about a wide variety of medications, procedures, etc.
* may not have the chance to gain in-depth knowledge about any one illness or condition
* may not have the opportunity to gain proficiency in some procedures, as do not perform them frequently

General nursing may be for you if:
- * you are a new graduate or want to gain a wide knowledge base
- * you enjoy working with a diverse group of patients

General nursing may *not* be for you if:
- * you prefer to learn in-depth about one type of patient or illness
- * you prefer the consistency of working with one type of patient, rather than a wide variety

Other factors to consider:
- * If you are new to a hospital, general floor nursing is a great way to become familiar with policies and procedures, how departments are run, and the physical layout of the hospital.

* * * * * * * * * * * * * * * * * * * * * *

Personal notes/comments:

## SPECIALTY AREA

Pros:
- * gain "in-depth" knowledge about a specific area; become an expert in a certain area
- * become proficient at specialized skills, knowledgeable about medications, monitors, and procedures pertaining to the specialty area
- * may work on a "closed" unit, where you are not required to float
- * may work with the same nurses and doctors almost every day

Cons:
- * may lose proficiency at skills you don't use often
- * may work with the same nurses and doctors every day
- * may get bored if you are not challenged with something new every day

A specialty area may be for you if:
*   you enjoy learning in-depth about any one illness, disease, or type of patient
*   you enjoy working with the same people almost every day

A specialty area may *not* be for you if:
*   you get bored doing the same thing every day
*   you like to use many different nursing skills

Other factors to consider:
*   Before you transfer to, or choose a specialty area, carefully consider the personalities of the people you will be working with and the dynamics of the unit you choose. You may choose to work in a specialty area part-time to gain a sense of the dynamics of the unit.

    To work in a specialty area, you may have to take classes (usually provided by the hospital, and you are usually paid for attending the classes). You may have to show proficiency in certain skills periodically (ACLS, PALS, etc.) Again, this re-certification is usually provided by the hospital.

\* \* \* \* \* \* \* \* \* \* \* \* \* \* \* \* \* \* \* \*

Personal notes/comments:

## DETERMINING YOUR PREFERENCE—
## GENERAL NURSING OR A SPECIALTY AREA

List the most important factors, regarding your career, which will help you determine whether you prefer to work in a general or specialty area (Examples: new graduate, desire to gain specialty certification)

From the information in this chapter, and your own personal assessment of needs and goals, would you prefer (circle one):

General nursing               Specialty area

**Transfer this answer to the "My Perfect Job" worksheet on page 174 of this book.

* * * * * * * * * * * * * * * * * * * *

## PRIMARY OR TEAM NURSING?

In primary nursing, each nurse is responsible for his or her own patients. In team nursing, an RN Team Leader may be responsible for several other RN's or LPN's as well as their patients. S/he may or may not be assigned patients. The Team Leader RN supervises other nurses, acts as a resource person, and does treatments and procedures that other personnel are not licensed or qualified to do; IV's for example. The Team Leader may make calls to the lab, pharmacy, doctors, etc., for the other nurses on the team. The Team Leader is responsible, in most cases, for the care given by the other nurses on the team. Responsibilities may vary according to facility policy.

## PRIMARY NURSING

In facilities using primary nursing, a nurse (RN or LPN) is responsible for his or her own patients, with a Head Nurse or Charge Nurse supervising the floor or area.

Pros:
   *    a primary care nurse provides total care for her patients
   *    opportunity to develop close relationships with patients

Cons:
   *    may not know anything about other patients on the floor, yet be asked to monitor and assist them when other nurses take breaks
   *    may be hard to find someone to help you lift or transfer a patient or assist with unfamiliar or difficult procedures
   *    responsible for complete patient care, including telephone calls, talking with doctors and the family, etc.

Primary care nursing may be for you if:
   *    you like direct patient care
   *    you enjoy being responsible for all aspects of patient care

Primary care nursing may *not* be for you if:
   *    you would rather supervise patient care (as a Team Leader, Head Nurse, Charge Nurse)

*   you prefer to have a resource person available to help you and answer any questions

Other factors to consider:

*   As a primary care nurse, you communicate directly with your patients' doctors. This alleviates any misunderstandings that may occur when orders go through your Team Leader, when you are a Team Member.

    As a primary care nurse, you know exactly what has, and has not been done. If you are a Team Leader, you must depend on Team Member reports to determine what has and has not been done.

\* \* \* \* \* \* \* \* \* \* \* \* \* \* \* \* \* \* \* \*

Personal notes/comments:

## TEAM NURSING—TEAM LEADER

Pros:

*   usually do not perform routine tasks such as bathing, medication administration
*   may perform, or assist with, challenging procedures

Cons:

*   may be in charge of many patients, incompetent nurses, etc.

Team nursing—as a Team Leader—may be for you if:

*   you don't mind making phone calls
*   you are comfortable supervising others
*   you are willing and able to teach other nurses about medications, treatments, and other aspects of patient care
*   you have good organizational and assessment skills and can set priorities and help other nurses set priorities
*   you do not enjoy routine "hands on" nursing

Team nursing—as a Team Leader—may *not* be for you if:
* you do not like to be in charge of other nurses
* you prefer "hands on" care and close contact with patients
* you are a new graduate, as you must be proficient at—and comfortable with—all aspects of patient care

Other factors to consider:
* A Team Leader must be proficient in all aspects of patient care. S/he must be comfortable assigning tasks and teaching other nurses. As you become acquainted with your team members' abilities, Team Leading will be easier as you'll become familiar with team members strengths and weaknesses.

* * * * * * * * * * * * * * * * * * * * *

Personal notes/comments:

## TEAM NURSING—TEAM MEMBER

Being a Team Member is much like primary care nursing. A definite advantage is having your Team Leader as a resource person who can double check assessment findings, assist with unfamiliar or difficult procedures, and make phone calls for you.

Pros:
* provide hands-on nursing care
* resource person (Team Leader) can answer questions, double check assessment findings, assist with lifting, transferring, unfamiliar or difficult procedures, and/or make phone calls to the doctor, family, lab, pharmacy, etc.

Cons:
* Team Leader may ask you to provide patient care in the way s/he prefers
* if you are not comfortable with your Team Leader you may have conflicts regarding patient care

45

Team nursing—as a Team Member—might be for you if:
* you are a new graduate, or new to a specific clinical area and feel more comfortable with a resource person

Team nursing—as a Team Member—might *not* be for you if:
* you prefer to work independently

Other factors to consider:
* If you are an RN, or an LPN planning to become an RN, you may start out as a Team Member and eventually be assigned as a Team Leader.

* * * * * * * * * * * * * * * * * * * *

Personal notes/comments:

## DETERMINING PRIMARY OR TEAM NURSING

List your most important career needs and goals related to your preference for team or primary nursing: (Example: new graduate, experienced nurse looking for a new challenge)

\* \* \* \* \* \* \* \* \* \* \* \* \* \* \* \* \* \* \* \*

From the information on the previous pages, do you prefer Team Nursing or Primary Care?

Primary care          Team nursing

Transfer your answer to the "My Perfect Job" worksheet on page 174 of this book.

\* \* \* \* \* \* \* \* \* \* \* \* \* \* \* \* \* \* \* \*

# What Are Your Strengths?
## Skills Checklists

*"Look at your own strengths and weaknesses and use these to find out what you are suited for."* Dee Dee Logue, RN

A nurse must have many skills, not only to provide good patient care, but also to get along with other nurses, doctors, hospital employees, as well as patients and their families.

We have divided nursing skills into four areas; Technical, Interpersonal, Leadership, and Management. The following checklists will help you assess the skills at which you are proficient, and those in which you need more experience or training. After each skill listed, make a check in the "yes" column if you are comfortable performing the skill without supervision; "no" if regardless of training or experience, you do *not* want to use this skill in your Perfect Job; and "willing to learn" if you need additional supervision or training to perform the skill, *and* are willing to undergo that training.

If you are a new graduate, you may not have actually performed many of the skills listed. Base your answers on skills you performed during clinical rotations. Some answers may also be based on observations, and others on skills you think you might want to use in your Perfect Job. Your answers may change over time, after you have actual experience with more of the skills listed. Thats OK—it means your Target Area is being narrowed down.

If you have worked as a nurse for some time, you may be able to fill out the majority of the Skills Checklist based on your experiences.

After each of the job descriptions in Section Two, there is a brief description of skills (Technical, Interpersonal, Leadership, and/or Management) which are very important in performing the job listed. There is also a Comprehensive Skills List, which lists skills needed for each job, at the end of Section Two.

If you are proficient in many skills in one of the following areas, or willing to learn the skills listed, you may consider a job which requires proficiency in this area. If you do not enjoy performing skills in any given area, or are not willing to learn these skills, you will not be happy in a job which requires these skills.

# TECHNICAL SKILLS

Technical skills are "hands on" skills that can range from very basic (giving oral medications), to extremely complex (titrating IV cardiac medications; ie. mcg/kg/m="x" cc/hour). Every job requires knowledge of technical skills.

| SKILL | YES | NO | WILLING TO LEARN |
|---|---|---|---|
| Basic IV skills (inserting, maintaining, continuous infusions) | | | |
| Advanced IV skills (Groshongs, Infus-a-ports, PCA pumps, central lines, PICC lines, TPN) | | | |
| Basic medication administration (oral, intramuscular, rectal, sublingual, subcutaneous, by NG/gastrostomy tube) | | | |
| Advanced medication administration (IV, PCA pump, endotracheal, chemotherapy), | | | |
| Basic monitoring (vital signs, general assessment, uncomplicated wounds). | | | |
| Advanced monitoring (CVP lines, telemetry, Swan-Ganz, arterial, right and left atrial pressure lines, post-partum). | | | |
| Basic lab specimens (obtaining urine and stool specimens, venous blood draws, wound cultures) and knowledge of what results will require the physicians' immediate attention. | | | |

Advanced lab specimens (obtaining
blood from central lines, Groshongs,
Infus-a-ports; assisting with
bladder and spinal taps; arterial
blood draws) and knowledge of what
results require the physician's
immediate attention

Basic post-surgical assessments
(vital signs, airway patency,
dressing condition and later wound
assessment, I & O, need for
analgesics, motor, sensation
and circulation assessment)

Advanced post-surgical assessments
(managing intubated patients, chest
tubes, pulse oximeters, Swan-Ganz
and arterial lines, etc.)

Basic patient education (hospital
routine, vital signs, medications,
discharge instructions)

Advanced patient education (complex
surgical procedures, complex
medication routines including drug
incompatibilities and drug precautions)

Basic procedures (simple dressing
changes, measuring I & O, inserting
a Foley catheter, admitting and
discharging patients, basic CPR)

Advanced procedures (complicated
dressing changes, assisting with
cardiac, GI, or respiratory procedures,
Code procedures)

## INTERPERSONAL SKILLS

Interacting with other people—nurses, doctors, people from other departments, and let's not forget our patients and their families—requires interpersonal skills. These skills are often known as "people skills", and are those necessary for dealing with—you guessed it—other people. A "people person" is a person who can deal effectively and calmly with difficult doctors, nasty nurses, impatient patients, and frantic families.

Interpersonal communication requires more than just the ability to articulate well. It also involves assuring the correct perception of the message you sent—for example, having the patient verbalize his understanding of the information you just presented to him.

Interpersonal skills are difficult to measure. Most of the time they are gained and perfected through practice.

| SKILL | YES | NO | WILLING TO LEARN |
|---|---|---|---|
| Routine communication with nurses, doctors, people from other departments | | | |
| Routine communication with patients and families | | | |
| Communicating with angry, or difficult-to-deal-with, doctors, nurses, people from other departments | | | |
| Communicating with angry, frantic, non-compliant, etc. patients and families | | | |
| Communicating with patients who have psychiatric diagnosis; depression, schizophrenia, etc. | | | |
| Being assertive with doctors, nurses (insisting on a medication change when the patient is having adverse effects—being a patient advocate) | | | |

Modifying usual hospital routines
per patient/family request (bathing
a patient after lunch, allowing a
patient to sleep through a poorly
timed treatment)

Accepting criticism; talking with
the person at a later time if it
was inappropriate

## *LEADERSHIP/SUPERVISORY SKILLS*

Leadership can be defined as actions that assist members of a group to achieve certain goals. For the purposes of this book, a nurse in a position of leadership is a Charge Nurse or Head Nurse, in charge of other nurses and ancillary personnel making up the nursing department (nurses aids, etc). The goal of the group, of course, is to provide good, safe, patient care.

Part of being a leader is leading in such a way that the other members of the group are willing to accept this leadership. Leading involves setting goals, dealing with conflicts, and disciplining if necessary. A nurse in a leadership position must be proficient in both technical and interpersonal skills.

| SKILL | YES | NO | WILLING TO LEARN |
|---|---|---|---|
| Ablity to supervise other nurses and assure necessary tasks are done (patient care) | | | |
| Making patient assignments to people qualified to perform the duties and procedures delegated to them | | | |
| Setting priorities with patient care, personnel issues, supervisory issues | | | |

Able to gain the cooperation of
of nursing personnel in meeting
standards of good patient care

Organizing time to get highest
priority tasks done

Troubleshooting and problem
solving (equipment, patients
and family, staff conflicts)

Mediating and diffusing conflicts
between staff, staff and patients
and/or family, and patients and
family members

Referring staff members to
management when necessary,
with patience and tact

## MANAGEMENT SKILLS

For the purposes of this book, a manager is a Director of Nursing, Assistant Director of Nursing, or House Supervisor. These managers do not do direct patient care except in unusual circumstances. However, managers must be proficient in technical, interpersonal, and leadership skills, as they are resource people for other nurses dealing with difficult or unusual circumstances (an angry doctor, Code situations, etc.)

**SKILL**                                    **YES   NO   WILLING TO LEARN**

Dealing with staff members having
personal problems

Willingness to confront and follow
up on sensitive issues such as
suspected addiction, patient
abuse or neglect, etc., by nurses,
doctors, or other hospital personnel

Following proper procedures and
completing "paper trail" when
dealing with difficult nurses,
doctors, other personnel or
other departments, as above

Willing to confront and solve
problems involving other
departments

Proficient at, or can successfully
delegate scheduling, Care Plans,
Infection Control, chart reviews,
and other tasks

Comfortable being a *nurse* advocate;
asking for more staff, higher wages,
better benefits, and so on

Willing to plan and work on long
term projects; new charting system,
changing from 8 to 12 hour
shifts, etc.

Knowledge, ability, and willingness
to be aware of and follow local,
state and federal regulations
regarding patient care, Care Plans,
patient rights, continuing
education (staff members), and so on

Willingness and ability to attend
numerous meetings and serve on (or
be in charge of!) various committees.

Ability to work with administrative
personnel (hospital or nursing home
administrator, president, hospital
board), who may have no concept
of what nursing care really is.

Willing to be "on call" virtually 24 hours
a day, and willing and able to perform
any and all duties of anyone supervised.

* * * * * * * * * * * * * * * * * * *

Personal notes/comments:

*"Get out there and try! Regardless of the area, you're increasing your skills that will make you a more caring nurse."* Teressa Williams, R.N.

# SKILLS CHECKLIST EVALUATION

*"A nurse must be efficient, knowledgeable, flexible, and deliver good patient care."* Bev Bergum, RN

List the most important factors, that will determine which skills you want to use in Your Perfect Job. (Examples: do *not* enjoy delegating, enjoy the challenge of difficult situations, enjoy learning and using new technical skills)

From the answers above, complete the following: Skill(s) I prefer to use in my Perfect Job:

Technical                                 Interpersonal

    Leadership                          Management

Transfer your answer(s) to the My Perfect Job Worksheet on page 174 of this book.

Transfer your answer(s) to the My Perfect Job Worksheet on page 174 of this book.

\* \* \* \* \* \* \* \* \* \* \* \* \* \* \* \* \* \* \* \*

# Interest Assessment

You've determined many specific characteristics for your Perfect Job. You have decided whether you want to work part-time or full-time, in a small or large facility, as a primary nurse or as part of a team. Now it's time to look at characteristics of the specific area of nursing in which you may choose to work.

Even though this is the last chapter of this section, your honest and well-thought out answers are every bit as important as those in the previous chapters, so take your time!

As you consider the answers to the following questions, think back upon clinical and work experiences.

Of your past jobs and/or clinical experiences, which did you enjoy the most? (Do *not* consider the facility itself or the people you worked with; consider the *nursing* aspects of the job only)

What, *specifically* did you enjoy about these areas of nursing? (Examples: age of patients, using hands-on skills, working independently, supporting family members) Again, consider *only* the nursing aspects of the job.

Of clinical areas and/or past jobs, which did you *dislike* the most?

What, *specifically,* did you *dislike* about the areas? (nursing aspects only) (Examples: many patients died, age of the patients, little patient contact)

\* \* \* \* \*

Now that you have looked at nursing aspects of past jobs and experiences, let's evaluate facility and co-worker factors.

Of clinical experiences and past jobs you enjoyed, what, specifically, did you enjoy about the facility and the people you worked with?
(Exmaples: new facility, up-to-date equipment, supportive administration, co-workers friendly and knowledgeable)

Of experiences and jobs you did *not* enjoy, list specific dislikes related to the facility itself, and the people you worked with. (Examples:
equipment very outdated, supervisors not efficient, co-workers not
supportive, facility often dirty)

\* \* \* \* \*

Obviously, you can't control or predict all aspects of a job. *Every*
facility has problems, and in *every* job there will be people with
whom you do not enjoy working. However, by being aware of factors
that influence your job satisfaction, you can observe for, and ask
questions to elicit at least *some* of this information. More suggestions
appear in Section Three, "Making the Interview Work for You."

# SECTION TWO

# Where Do I Belong?
# What Are My Options?
# Choosing The Area For
# Your Perfect Job

*"Look, look, look."* Donna Nickel, RN

# How to Use This Section

This section lists many of the areas in which a nurse has the option to work. We have given you a list of general duties of each area, pros and cons of working in the area, and thoughts as to why this area may, or might not, be for you.

Please keep in mind these are only guidelines, and a nurse's duties and responsibilities may be very different from facility to facility.

We have also given you information about skills required for these jobs. Most facilities will offer training and education necessary to perform the specialty skills necessary to that particular area. However, if you are not interested in learning these skills, or even if you are proficient at these skills, if you are not interested in using them, you should consider a different clinical area. A "Skills Utilization Checklist," at the end of Section Two, summarizes skills used in each job.

We have also provided space for "Personal notes/comments." Use this area to jot down any thoughts about that specific area—perhaps the name of someone who is working in that area, who you could use as a resource person.

You may choose to read straight through this section, or begin with areas you have worked in or think you might like to work in, and skip around. Either way is OK, but don't rule out working in a particular area until you've read about it—you may find that an area that didn't appeal to you actually fits your Perfect Job description!

As you read through this section, fill in the worksheet at the end of this section, "Interest List: Areas in Which I Have *Some* Interest; Areas in Which I have a *Strong* Interest." Even if a job in a particular area is not realistic for you at this time, it may be in the future.

When you see an ad, or hear about a job opening in a specific area on your Interest List, review the information regarding that area. Before your interview, jot down specific questions about that area of nursing.

The information was provided by nurses who have worked, or currently are working, in the area being discussed.

*"Go into each clinical area with your eyes open. Get rid of any pre-conceived ideas regarding that area."* Terry Lahnstein, R.N.

# Direct Patient Care Areas
## *In-Hospital*

## Medical/Surgical—General Floor Nursing

Medical/Surgical (med/surg) nursing is often referred to as "floor nursing." Med/surg nurses care for medical patients, who may have such diversified diagnoses as decubitus ulcers, blood clots, bladder infection or other medical diagnosis; or surgical patients, who return to the floor after an appendectomy, cholecystectomy, amputation, etc.

Med/surg nurses usually care for six or more patients at a time, and are responsible for the patient's Activities of Daily Living (ADL's), medications, treatments, and procedures ordered during the nurse's shift. The nurse must be very organized to complete each assigned patient's care, as some patients may be off the floor during the shift having tests or other treatments or procedures done. The nurse may spend valuable patient-care time on the telephone talking with doctors, or scheduling tests, procedures, and special treatments.

Specialized med/surg units are discussed in the following chapter.

Pros:
*   gain knowledge about a wide variety of illnesses and diseases including their treatments, medications, procedures, as well as lab tests and their implications
*   exposure to a variety of medications, procedures, treatments
*   good patient continuity, as many med/surg patients spend several days or more in the hospital
*   the nurse is influential in planning and implementing patient care
*   use different technical skills every day

Cons:
*   patient load may be heavy
*   physical work; lifting, transferring, turning patients, etc.
*   may experience burn-out due to heavy patient load and caring for the same chronic patients over a long period of time
*   may not do some treatments and procedures frequently enough to feel comfortable doing them

* difficult to meet all patient and family members' needs while completing work assignment
* paperwork and charting

This area may be for you if:
* you are a new graduate, as you will gain experience giving medications, performing procedures and treatments
* you are a new graduate or have not found an area of nursing you really enjoy, as you will be exposed to many different types of patients and may determine a specific area of interest
* you would like to gain a wide base of knowledge about a variety of illnesses, medications, procedures, treatments, lab tests and their implications
* you like to use many different nursing skills on a daily basis
* you like working with a variety of patients
* you enjoy working with long-term patients and their families
* you are well organized

This area may *not* be for you if:
* you don't like to or are unable to lift, turn, or transfer patients
* you have trouble organizing your day
* you like to know, before you come to work, the type of patients you will be caring for
* you would rather gain specialized knowledge about specific diseases, patients, or conditions

Other information to consider:
Med/surg is a great place to gain experience if you are a new graduate or have not worked in hospital nursing for awhile. With the wide variety of patients you will work with and the many skills you use, you may find a type of procedure you enjoy performing, or certain patients you enjoy caring for, which may help you decide on a specialty area which is fulfilling to you.

Skills needed:
* knowledge of, and the ability to perform basic technical skills; medication administration, IV's, dressing changes, catheter insertion and care, interpretation of lab results
* technical skills; the ability to assess the whole patient, with a general understanding of the specific body system affected by the illness or disease

62

* good interpersonal skills for dealing with doctors, people from other departments, family members
* willingness to learn

* * * * * * * * * * * * * * * * * * * * *

Personal notes/comments:




# Medical/Surgical—Specialty Floor Nursing

Medical/surgical (med/surg) specialty units include orthopedics, gynecology, neurology, telemetry, oncology, etc., in which patients with one specific diagnosis, or problems primarily affecting just one body system, are treated.

See Medical/Surgical—General Floor Nursing for more information.

Pros:
* gain knowledge of, and proficiency in, specialized treatments, medications, procedures, and lab tests necessary to treat patients with a narrow range of problems
* learn specialty skills and procedures
* opportunity to use specialized technical skills on a daily basis

Cons:
* little variety in patient problems and diagnoses
* much physical work; lifting, turning, transferring patients
* *may* have a heavy patient load
* lots of paperwork and charting

This area may be for you if:
* you want to gain knowledge of, and proficiency at, treating patients with a narrow range of diagnoses
* you are willing to learn specialized procedures

* you like to know, before coming to work, what type of patients you will be caring for

This area may *not* be for you if:
* you would rather have a wide base of knowledge about illnesses, treatments, lab tests, procedures, etc.
* you get bored working with the same type of patient daily
* you are a new graduate, as you will *not* be gaining a wide base of knowledge and experience

Other information about this area:
Consider working on a specialty unit part time before making a permanent commitment to working in an area that may or may not be for you!

Skills needed:
* wide range of basic assessment and technical skills, along with specialty skills related to the area
* see Med/Surg—General Floor Nursing for more information

* * * * * * * * * * * * * * * * * * * * *

Personal notes/comments:

# Out-Patient Services

Out-patient Services (OPS) is an in-facility department whose patients are routinely sent home after surgery or treatment (patients *are* admitted if complications occur).
OPS offers services such as; surgeries (tonsillectomies, hernia repair), blood transfusions, IV therapy (including antibiotics), and chemotherapy, in many facilities.
Nurses are required to do a lot of teaching, regarding the procedure itself, follow-up care, and any medications prescribed.

OPS departments are open day hours, although those hours may be 5 AM - 8 PM. A nurse may be required to stay later to care for patients who cannot be discharged until later in the evening. OPS is one of the fastest-growing areas in health- care today.

Pros:
* fast pace, never boring!
* work with a wide variety of patients of different ages and with different diagnoses and procedures performed
* patients are usually happy, as they return home the same day
* "serial patients"—those who return routinely for chemotherapy, IV antibiotics, etc., become familiar to you
* opportunity to work one-to-one with patients during frequent assessments required
* easy to leave your job at work

Cons:
* some doctors may expect the nurse to know what his orders are and expect nurses to follow *his* policies, regardless of written orders or facility policy
* patients who arrive with no doctor's orders
* don't get to develop close or long-term relationship with most patients
* may have to stay past "closing time" with patients who are not sufficiently recovered to go home

This area may be for you if:
* you have good assessment skills and a strong med/surg background
* you can recognize surgical complications and difficulties; for example, allergies to medication that the patient did not state
* you are organized and can work at a fast pace while prioritizing patient needs
* you have good teaching skills
* you have excellent interpersonal skills for dealing with patients, families, and doctors
* you can encourage patients to get up, urinate, take fluids, etc. (requirements for dismissal)
* you are willing to take classes or undergo training necessary to perform certain skills (LPN's must have additional training to work with IV's)

This area may *not* be for you if:
*   you are a new graduate, as you do not yet have the compre-
    hensive assessment skills necessary for working with
    short-term patients
*   you would rather develop a closer relationship with your pa-
    tients
*   you do not enjoy the fast pace and fast turn-over of patients
    in this area

Other information about this area:
A nurse working in OPS must have multiple skills necessary to
admit, assess, teach, recover, and dismiss patients within a very short
period of time. Experience is needed to learn the right questions to
ask, and to spot subtle signs of post-op complications.

Skills needed:
*   assessment skills to obtain an accurate history and physical
    prior to surgery, and assess pain, respiratory function, wound
    condition, etc., after surgery is completed
*   ability to teach pre-op information, at-home cares, signs and
    symptoms to report, etc.
*   ability to teach patients and caregivers of various education
    and comprehension levels
*   interpersonal skills to deal tactfully with doctors
*   interpersonal skills to deal with patients and families if
    surgery is delayed or the patient has to stay over night due to
    complications or problems
*   organizational skills to deal with numerous patients in any
    phase of pre-op, post-op, ready to be dismissed, etc.

* * * * * * * * * * * * * * * * * * * * * *

Personal notes/comments:

# Emergency Room (ER)

An Emergency Room (ER) is staffed with several nurses, (usually RN's) doctors, and occasionally Nurse Practitioners, Emergency Medical Technician's (EMT's) or paramedics, in large facilities. ER doctors may rotate ER duty or work in the ER permanently. In small hospitals, the doctor may have to be called in when an emergency patient arrives in the ER.

The ER nurse triages patients, takes the patient to an exam room, does a basic assessment, notifies the ER doctor, and carries out the doctor's orders.

Pros:
* patient care is very short term; most patients spend several hours or less in the ER
* use a variety of technical skills
* learn about emergency drugs and a wide variety of procedures
* work with a large variety of age groups
* become familiar with numerous community services; ambulance, police, mental health, etc.

Cons:
* patient contact is short term and often you don't know the outcome of the patient's condition after s/he leaves the ER
* some patients abuse the system and you may see them often for minor or insignificant complaints

This area may be for you if:
* you can think on your feet and enjoy the fast-paced activities of true emergency situations
* you like a quickly changing patient load
* you enjoy working with a wide variety of patients of different ages
* you have good basic nursing knowledge so you can assist with a wide variety of different patients; for example, prepping a patient for a heart catheterization in one room, and assisting with the reduction of a fracture in the next
* you don't mind not knowing what your next patient's illness or injury will be

This area may *not* be for you if:
- * you have limited knowledge of basic care for different age groups and diagnoses
- * you have poor organizational skills
- * you don't like the uncertainty of not knowing what the patient, or day, will bring
- * you don't enjoy crisis situations
- * you have difficulty leaving work at work (there are very sad, unpleasant experiences)

Other information to consider:

ER nurses are usually required to be certified in Advanced Cardiac Life Support (ACLS) and Pediatric Advanced Life Support (PALS).

Skills needed:
- * the ability to do a good, complete assessment, and ask pertinent questions about the presenting complaint or problem
- * good technical skills for all age groups; IV's, injections, giving medications, reading EKG's, CPR
- * good interpersonal skills for dealing with a multitude of personalities and situations—hysterical or grieving family members, difficult ancillary department staff with whom you need to coordinate patient care (i.e. X-ray department, lab, pharmacy, etc.)

* * * * * * * * * * * * * * * * * * * *

Personal notes/comments:

# Operating Room

An Operating Room (O.R.) Nurse cares for the patient immediately before, and during surgery. The scrub nurse is "sterile" during surgery, and assists the doctor with the surgical procedure; handing instruments, positioning the patient, etc. The circulating nurse coordinates all O.R. activities, and manages and documents all nursing aspects of the patient's OR time and is accountable for assuring presence of all instruments, sponges, and so on at the end of the case.

Pros:
* wear scrubs provided by and/or laundered by the hospital
* learn and use specialized technical skills
* develop a close relationship with the doctors, anesthesiologists, and other nurses
* work in a very clean environment

Cons:
* little patient and/or family contact
* operations may be long, requiring standing for hours
* may work with difficult or demanding doctors
* may not know patient outcome after s/he leaves surgery

This area may be for you if:
* you can work well under pressure
* you have good dexterity and are mechanically inclined, as you work with many instruments and machines
* you prefer short term patient contact
* you do not enjoy a lot of patient and family contact
* you can work closely with a team of nurses, doctors, the anesthesiologist, etc.
* you can tactfully inform doctors or other personnel of breaks in sterile technique

This area may *not* be for you if:
* you have many family or outside commitments, as "on-call" hours may be required
* you enjoy patient contact
* you do not enjoy working with doctors, anesthesiologists, etc. constantly

* you are claustrophobic, as masks, gowns, etc., can be restrictive

Other information to consider:
In a small hospital, there may only be one shift and the OR nurses may be required to work the whole shift, regardless of extended hours.

Skills needed:
* basic assessment skills when evaluating the patient before and during surgery
* technical skills related to preparing the patient for surgery and assuring patient safety during surgery (positioning, monitoring vital signs)
* ability to care for the patient amid all the activity of O.R.
* knowledge of and the ability to observe sterile techniques, policies and procedures related to the O.R.
* technical skills when working with instruments and other OR equipment
* good interpersonal skills when dealing with difficult doctors, staff members, patients, and family members
* the ability to teach patients and new O.R. personnel

* * * * * * * * * * * * * * * * * * * * * *

Personal notes/comments:

# Recovery Room (RR)/
# Post Anesthesia Care Unit (PACU)

Recovery Room/Post Anesthesia Care nurses care for patients immediately after surgery, until they have recovered sufficiently from anesthesia and can go to their room or ICU. As well as assessing the patient's recovery, the nurse may report the patient's condition to family members. A recovery nurse may be required to be "on-call" and available to return to the hospital on nights, weekends, and/or holidays, if someone needs emergency surgery.

Pros:
*   "on-call" pay may be time-and-a-half or double regular pay
*   a variety of shifts may be available; 6 AM-2 PM, 7 AM - 3 PM, 8 AM - 4 PM, etc.
*   fast paced, rapid turnover of patients
*   use many technical and assessment skills with each patient

Cons:
*   patient's condition may change very rapidly
*   if the patient is discharged to the floor at night it may be difficult to find help for the transfer
*   "on-call" status can be difficult if you are called in the middle of the night or when personal plans are interrupted
*   may be difficult to find child care to cover long shifts and "on-call" hours
*   very little contact with a conscious, oriented, patient

Recovery nursing may be for you if:
*   you enjoy a fast paced environment
*   you enjoy using specialized technical skills
*   you are comfortable with, and can act quickly and appropriately in, a crisis situation
*   you don't mind unpredictable and "on-call" hours

Recovery nursing may *not* be for you if:
*   you have small children and don't have reliable sitters for "on-call" situations
*   you enjoy developing a relationship with your patients
*   you don't like to use highly technical skills
*   you don't enjoy frequent monitoring and assessment of patients

Other information to consider:
    Small hospitals may have just one regular shift for recovery nurses; these nurses may be required to work overtime if surgeries last longer than expected, or a patient is not ready to be transferred out of the Recovery Room at the end of the shift.

Skills needed:
*   excellent assessment skills with regards to airway, circulation, wounds, bleeding, pain, movement, sensation, etc.
*   variety of technical skills related to airway management; working with intubated patients on ventilators or T-pieces, oxygen delivery systems, pulse oximeters, various monitors
*   interpersonal skills; the ability to clearly explain to family members the process of recovery, and the reasons recovery may be longer than initially expected

* * * * * * * * * * * * * * * * * * * * *

Personal notes/comments:

# Critical Care/Intensive Care Unit/ Post-Intensive Care Unit

Critical Care(CC)/Intensive Care Unit (ICU) nursing involves specialized care for critically ill patients. Patients in ICU may be in the process of having a heart attack, recovering after open heart or other major surgery, or have other life-threatening medical or surgical complications requiring close monitoring with highly technical equipment. They usually have complex medication routines and require complicated procedures. Specialized ICU's may care for neonatal, pediatric, or cardiac patients, to name a few.

The environment is professional and fast paced. An ICU nurse must be able to anticipate changes in his or her patients and make immediate decisions based upon these changes.

ICU's are usually staffed by RN's, although facility policy may also allow LPN's with IV training to work there. An ICU nurse usually has one to three patients assigned to her; however, most patients in ICU require total care and almost constant assessment, as well as frequent interventions. When patients do not need the close monitoring of ICU, they may be transferred to a general floor or to the Post Intensive Care Unit (PICU). On the PICU, patients still require frequent monitoring, but are considered more stable. A nurse may care for a greater number of patients on the PICU.

Pros:
* low nurse to patient ratio
* learn about new procedures, techniques, medications, and equipment
* utilize *many* advanced technical skills
* able to see changes in patients (good *and* bad), usually rapidly
* other staff members usually very well qualified and trained
* good continuity of care due to low nurse/patient ratio

Cons:
* may be floated to other units when census is low, and given difficult patients and/or a heavy patient load as ICU nurses are considered "supernurses"
* can be very stressful, especially if you are new to the specialty area and unsure of your abilities
* stressful to deal with the families of critically ill patients

This area may be for you if:
* you enjoy a fast-paced, challenging environment
* you enjoy learning about new techniques, equipment, procedures, medications
* you enjoy working with just a few patients
* you want to use technical skills and learn new skills
* you have very good assessment skills

This area may *not* be for you if:
* you do not enjoy working in a stressful environment
* you do not enjoy total patient care or direct patient care
* you see illness as depressing; patients do not go home from ICU; they get transferred to another floor when they improve
* you are not confident you have the necessary skills to work in ICU, or are not willing to learn these skills

Other information to consider:
ICU/PICU nursing will keep your mind challenged with the new developments that occur almost daily. A new graduate should have some experience and be comfortable with standard procedures (IV's, medication administration) before working in the ICU.

A nurse with a special interest in Critical Care may obtain certification in this specialty and become a CCRN (Critical Care Registered Nurse).

Skills needed:
* a wide variety of technical skills; interpreting monitor readings (oximeter, telemetry), lab results and their implications, working with highly technical equipment (ventilators, chest tubes, central lines), complex medication routines (titrated to blood pressure or pulse or calculated by patient weight), and advanced procedures (assisting with the insertion of central lines, chest tubes, pacemakers)
* excellent assessment techniques; the ICU nurse must be proficient at assessing all aspects of the patient and relating these findings to the disease process and potential complications
* good interpersonal skills in dealing with doctors and families of critically ill patients
* required to take classes and be up-to-date in Basic and Advanced Cardiac Life Support protocols

* * * * * * * * * * * * * * * * * * * * *

Personal notes/comments:

# Rehabilitation

Patients are received on a rehabilitation (rehab) area after their condition has stabilized following a stroke, head injury, or paralyzing accident. Patients enter a rehab area to relearn how to perform Activities of Daily Living (ADL's)—dressing, bathing, eating, etc.—to be as independent as possible after dismissal. Patients also learn at-home medical management of any diagnoses related to their injury; for example, many patients with paralysis must learn self-catheterization, others, how to follow their medication schedule.

Family members are often present much of the day, and must also be taught about the patient's condition and the necessary at-home cares.

Nurses must monitor patients overall conditions and be aware of and ready to treat any complications that may develop.

Nurses, Physical Therapists, Occupational Therapists, Speech Therapists, and tutors (for school-age patients) all work with patients who are undergoing rehab.

Pros:
*   patients are long-term, giving the nurse the opportunity to develop a professional relationship with them
*   fewer medical emergencies
*   generally a relaxed pace
*   very rewarding to see patients improving
*   there may be less charting than in other areas

Cons:
*   much physical work lifting and transferring patients
*   most patients will *not* regain all capabilities
*   many young patients
*   patients' progress may be very slow
*   may be difficult to schedule and work with ancillary departments (Physical Therapy, etc.)
*   patients may become depressed, angry, uncommunicative, etc.

This area may be for you if:
*   you like to work with long-term patients
*   you are able to do, and don't mind doing, a lot of physical work
*   you can encourage patients through the lengthy process of rehabilitation by pointing out small improvements
*   you have a lot of patience when teaching patients and families, and enjoy this type of teaching
*   you enjoy a relaxed pace of work

This area may *not* be for you if:
*   you want to use technical nursing skills daily
*   you like to see your patients progress quickly
*   you do not like, or cannot do, heavy physical activity

Other information to consider:

Teamwork is vital on rehab, as many patients require three or four nurses to turn, lift, and transfer them.

Skills needed:
* basic technical and assessment skills, with focus on positioning, transfers, and complications related to stroke, head injuries, and paralysis
* interpersonal skills to coordinate scheduling among other departments; for dealing with family members, and for helping the patient through depression, anger, etc.
* the ability to teach the patient and family members about the patient's condition and at-home cares required

* * * * * * * * * * * * * * * * * * * *

Personal notes/comments:

# Psychiatric

Psychiatric (psych) nurses care for patients with psychiatric diagnoses, which may include depression, eating disorders, drug or alcohol addiction, manic depression, and/or multiple personalities. Psychiatric units may care for children, adolescents, adults, or geriatric patients. A psychiatrist/psychologist monitors each patients progress and orders medications, labs, etc. when necessary. These doctors rely on the nurses' observations to gage their patients' progress. The psych nurse is responsible for monitoring a patient's physical health while working with the patient and health care team to improve the patient's mental health. Psych patients do not usually need technical procedures such as IV's or dressing changes.

Psych nurses may lead, or assist with group therapy sessions, and must enjoy communicating with patients beyond the usual "How are you feeling today?" Almost all patients need to be monitored for the potential to attempt suicide or harm themselves or others.

Pros:
* psych nurses usually wear street clothes
* infrequent lifting
* patients are usually hospitalized long-term, giving the nurse the opportunity to get to know them well
* although patients may have violent outbursts, the pace on psych units is usually slower than on other units

Cons:
* psych nursing can be mentally very stressful; patients may have sad, disturbing, violent histories
* it may take a long time for a patient to gain trust in nurses and therefore may take a long time for the nurse to see patient improvements
* patients may be manipulative, difficult to work with, non-compliant, and occasionally violent
* some patients do not improve, or are readmitted to the hospital numerous times, which can be discouraging for the nurse
* as the patients are long-term, it can be difficult for a nurse if a patient is antagonistic to her
* some nurses find charting behaviors, conversations, etc., more difficult than charting physical findings
* potential for injury to the employee if a resident has a violent outburst

This area may be for you if:
* you like to working with long-term patients
* you are a good listener and enjoy using therapeutic communication techniques
* you don't mind waiting a long time to see a patient improve
* you find difficult, uncooperative, unpredictable, manipulative, patients a challenge
* you are comfortable in unpredictable situations

This area may *not* be for you if:
* you enjoy performing technical procedures like IV's, NG's, dressings, and so on
* you like to see your patients get better fast
* you aren't comfortable dealing with a patients' feelings, emotions, and hearing about painful events/situations
* you are not comfortable confronting negative or inappropriate behaviors

* you are somewhat gullible and take patient behaviors personally

Other information to consider:

Basic psych communication skills are useful when dealing with *any* type of patient, and the nurse's own family! A psych nurse must be comfortable with herself, and be willing to confront her own feelings which may be brought out when working with psych patients.

Skills needed:
* interpersonal skills and therapeutic communication techniques to work with patients who may be angry, depressed, violent, manipulative, etc.
* technical skills—passing medications and monitoring for side effects

\* \* \* \* \* \* \* \* \* \* \* \* \* \* \* \* \* \* \* \*

Personal notes/comments:

# Labor and Delivery

A Labor and Delivery (L&D) nurse cares for the laboring woman from the time she enters the hospital through birth and recovery (about two hours after birth). L&D nurses must be very familiar with the stages of labor and delivery, and be prepared to deal with emergencies that can occur during the process. L&D nurses may care for high-risk moms-to-be, and newborns, too, in some hospitals. The L&D nurse may also care for patients in the hospital for pregnancy-related tests and procedures.

If a woman has had no prenatal care, she and her support person will need teaching and support throughout labor and delivery. Even if they have taken prenatal classes, they will need a review of the labor and delivery process, and support throughout it.

Pros:
* for the most part, a happy and fun area in which to work

* opportunity to develop and use specialized skills
* most patients are medically stable; the course of L&D is usually fairly predictable
* wear hospital scrubs, which may be provided and/or laundered by the hospital

Cons:
* responsible for two lives (mom and baby)
* emergencies occur suddenly and fast intervention is critical to the well-being of both mom and baby
* bad outcomes (fetal death) can be very difficult for the family, as well as the staff members involved

This area may be for you if:
* you enjoy working with families and being a part of a very special time in their lives
* you enjoy teaching
* you enjoy a fairly predictable routine

This area may *not* be for you if:
* you do not like potentially high-risk situations
* you don't enjoy teaching
* you are uncomfortable with non-traditional family situations (single mothers, teen-age mothers)

Other information to consider:
In some Labor and Delivery areas, the same nurse cares for the mother and baby from the time of birth until they are dismissed from the hospital.

Skills needed:
* technical skills needed when caring for a pregnant woman *not* in labor; assisting with amniocentesis; monitoring non-stress test and contraction stress tests (done to assess the well-being of the fetus)
* wide range of technical skills when caring for the laboring woman; assessing the Fetal Heart Rate (FHR), cervical dilation and effacement; length, strength, and frequency of contractions; the mother's vital signs; and carrying out doctor's orders which may include starting an IV, vaginal shave, and enema

* assist the mother with prepared childbirth techniques and support the mother as well as the support person throughout labor and delivery
* assess, and intervene appropriately, if maternal and/or fetal complications occur
* technical skills needed after delivery for new moms: frequent assessment of vital signs, vaginal bleeding, and the new mothers psychological response to birth
* good interpersonal skills to deal with a wide variety of family situations

* * * * * * * * * * * * * * * * * * * *

Personal notes/comments:

# Post-Partum

Post-partum care is the care of a woman from the time her baby is born until she is dismissed from the hospital. The mother is closely monitored for signs of excess bleeding and/or infection. She is instructed about bottle or breastfeeding and all other cares of the newborn, as well as the physical, mental, and emotional changes she will experience during the post-partum period.

The post-partum nurse must be prepared to deal with diverse family situations (single mothers, teen moms) and sad family situations (stillbirth, adoption, congenital defects, incest).

Women with post-partum complications, such as hemorrhage or infection, may be cared for on the post-partum unit or transferred to a specialty unit.

Pros:
* wear scrubs which may be provided by and/or laundered by the hospital
* one-to-one teaching of new moms
* short patient stay—usually one to two days after the baby is born
* usually a happy area

Cons:
* difficult to find time to teach as stay is so short
* can become boring as follow the same basic routine every day

This area may be for you if:
* you enjoy working with families
* you like to teach and are comfortable talking about breast-feeding, sexuality, etc.
* you prefer a fairly predictable routine
* you enjoy working with patients during a short stay
* you prefer to work with women patients

This area may *not* be for you if:
* you do not enjoy working with women
* you are not comfortable talking about body changes, breast-feeding, sexual issues, and lifestyle changes
* you find it difficult to accept lifestyle and parenting styles that you don't agree with
* you resent teenage mothers/single mothers
* you prefer to work with patients over a longer period of time

Other information to consider:
Physically caring for a mother who is post-partum may be routine, but the unusual situations your patients may have can challenge you as much—or more—than any physical problem!

Insurance companies are limiting a woman's stay in the hospital after the baby is born, and this will continue to be an issue.

Skills needed:
* good assessment and technical skills specific to the post-partum woman; assessing the woman's fundus, lochia, episiotomy, breasts
* excellent teaching skills about a variety of subjects, and the ability to teach women who have differing levels of education and comprehension
* interpersonal skills, especially when dealing with non-traditional family situations

* * * * * * * * * * * * * * * * * * * * *

81

Personal notes/comments:

# Newborn Nursery

Generally, newborns are cared for in the Newborn Nursery from birth until they are discharged from the hospital. Most hospitals now allow "rooming in" which (depending on facility policy) means that the baby is in his or her mother's room when she is awake, and in the nursery only at night or when the mother is sleeping or bathing, etc. Babies who are sick, or born with problems requiring close monitoring and frequent skilled treatments, will be admitted to a Neonatal Intensive Care Unit (NICU).

During their stay in the Newborn Nursery, babies are assessed by nurses and given a thorough examination by the physician who will be caring for the baby after dismissal. Nurses monitor the babies for any problems, feed the bottle- fed babies (if the mother is asleep), and carry out any doctor's orders.

Nursery nurses may teach new mothers about newborn care; bathing, feeding, circumcision care (when appropriate).

Pros:
* wear scrubs which may be provided by and/or laundered by the hospital
* usually a happy place to work
* few emergencies or crisis situations
* get to work with newborns

Cons:
* crying infants
* infants are usually dismissed one to two days after birth and it may be difficult to teach about all aspects of newborn care in this short time
* sad situations; newborn death, deformities or other problems with the baby

82

This area may be for you if:
* you enjoy caring for newborns
* you enjoy teaching about newborn care
* you are comfortable with non-traditional family situations (teen mothers, single mothers, etc.)
* you enjoy a relatively low stress working environment
* you enjoy having a fairly routine shift

This area may *not* be for you if:
* you enjoy conversing with your patients
* you are uncomfortable with non-traditional family situations
* you do not enjoy working with babies

Other information to consider:
   Nurses working in the Newborn Nursery are required to be certified in Pediatric Advanced Life Support (PALS). The certification and recertification are usually provided by the hospital.

Skills needed:
* technical skills specific to working with infants; routine orders may include Vitamin K shots (to prevent excess bleeding in the newborn), blood tests, (to screen for metabolic disorders) antibiotic eye drops, and Hepatitis B immunizations
* emergency technical skills that may be used include; starting an IV, administering oxygen, intubation, and transferring the baby to an NICU
* good interpersonal skills for teaching and working with mothers with varied educational levels and family situations

* * * * * * * * * * * * * * * * * * *

Personal notes/comments:

# Pediatrics

Pediatrics (peds) is the medical care of children under the age of 21 (although kids in their teens and older may be placed on an adult floor). Care includes prevention of problems (by teaching parents how to prevent illnesses and injuries), and treatment of children who are ill, preparing for, or recovering from surgery. Diagnoses may include; respiratory infection, broken bones, appendicitis, abuse, failure to thrive.

The pediatric nurse cares for the family as well as the patient, and must be able to teach caregivers how to do "at home" procedures—give medications, perform respiratory treatments, monitor signs and symptoms.

Pros:
* get to wear "fun" clothes—scrubs, lab jackets
* not much heavy lifting
* kids' conditions usually improve rapidly
* children are forgiving—even if a nurse must administer a painful procedure, the child will smile and hug him or her later
* peds area has a playful, relaxed, homelike atmosphere as much as possible

Cons:
* a patient may bring a lawsuit against the nurse or hospital until he or she is past the age of majority (state laws may vary)
* parents and patients may not understand the need for painful, although necessary, treatments
* very young patients are unable to verbalize needs, wants, pain levels, or other signs and symptoms
* many patients need almost one-to-one comforting and supervision; however, staffing does not allow this
* family situation may be dysfunctional—drug use and abuse, absent parents, mental, physical, or sexual abuse—and the nurse is obligated to be a patient advocate and report these situations, which can upset the parents
* patients may need total care with ADL's but be very uncooperative
* terminal illnesses and deaths are difficult to deal with

This area may be for you if:
* you enjoy working with children
* like to teach and work with families

This area may *not* be for you if:
* you need a strict routine to follow
* you are uncomfortable around children who are sick, crying, or in pain
* it is difficult for you to perform painful procedures on children
* you are uncomfortable confronting and dealing with situations that are potentially dangerous to a child; abuse, neglect, etc.

Other information to consider:
Visual and "hands on" assessments are very important as children may be unable to accurately communicate pain and other signs and symptoms. A pediatric nurse must be able to alter *his* or *her* routine to fit around her patients', as kids need to keep their home routine as much as possible while hospitalized.

Skills needed:
* very good assessment skills, and a variety of technical skills (IV's, medication administration, NG's, etc.), which must be adapted to working with pediatric patients
* interpersonal skills for dealing with patients, families, and doctors
* teaching skills; the ability to teach people with various levels of education and comprehension

* * * * * * * * * * * * * * * * * * * *

Personal notes/comments:

# Transplant

A transplant nurse is an RN who is required to be experienced in critical care nursing. S/he also must have the specialized training required for the particular transplant area in which s/he works—heart, lung, liver, kidney, etc.—for pediatric or adult patients. A nurse must be very skilled technically, and have excellent interpersonal skills, to care for transplant patients. Patients usually are transferred directly from surgery to the transplant floor, where they are recovered from anesthesia and remain for four to five days (barring complications), and then are transferred to a general floor.
(See Med/surg—specialty floor nursing for more information about specialized areas)

Pros:
*   very rewarding to see the rapid improvement of quality of life after a transplant is performed
*   gain proficiency in very specialized skills, and use them daily

Cons:
*   little variety in skills used and cares provided
*   due to reverse isolation techniques used, nurse may have very little contact with patients, only with other nurse s/he is working with in caring for the patient

This area may be for you if:
*   you have a strong background in Intensive Care
*   you enjoy learning and using specialized skills
*   you are able to, and enjoy, extensive patient and family teaching regarding medications, lifestyle changes, signs and symptoms to report to the doctor, etc.

This area may *not* be for you if:
*   you are a new graduate, as the knowledge and critical thinking this area requires comes only with experience
*   you do not want to develop and use specialized skills
*   you would rather work with a wider variety of patients

Other information to consider:
New graduates who would like to work on a transplant floor should begin by working on a Med/surg floor, to gain experience

with a wide variety of patients, procedures. etc. The nurse can then transfer to an Intensive Care area to develop and hone critical care skills, and then, when a position is available in a transplant area, apply for it!

Skills needed:
* advanced technical and assessment skills regarding recovering a patient from anesthesia, interpreting lab results, detecting infection and/or rejection, dressing changes, medication administration, reverse isolation procedures, etc.
* ability to teach patient and family members vital information regarding medications, signs and symptoms to report, lifestyle changes, etc.
* interpersonal skills to communicate with the patient and his or her family during this very stressful time

* * * * * * * * * * * * * * * * * * * * *

Personal notes/comments:

# Hemodialysis—Acute

Patients with acute kidney failure due to trauma or acute illness may be treated in the hospital, by a hemodialysis nurse. The pace will be quicker than in a Chronic Hemodialysis unit (see page 100), and dialysis may be done on an emergency basis.

Pros:
* learn and develop specialized technical skills

Cons:
* may require long hours (if many patients require dialysis), and may have "on-call" hours
* patients are acutely ill; may be stressful for the nurse

This area may be for you if:
- * you thrive on working in emergency situations
- * you like to work with critically ill patients, who may have multiple problems
- * you have excellent IV skills and enjoy using them
- * you enjoy interpreting lab values and adjusting treatment accordingly

This area may not be for you if:
- * you do not like working with acutely ill patients on an emergency basis

Other information to consider:
In the acute setting, the hemodialysis nurse will be working with a team of doctors and nurses to care for the critically ill patient.

Skills needed:
- * excellent assessment skills; of lab results, cardiac and respiratory status, fluid and electrolyte balance
- * technical skills; IV, mechanical (dialysis machine),
- * interpersonal skills to quickly develop a trusting relationship with patients and family members
- * to teach patient and family about the process of dialysis, implications of lab results and assessment findings

* * * * * * * * * * * * * * * * * * * * *

Personal notes/comments:

# Direct Patient Care Areas
## *Out-of-Hospital*

## Long Term Care (LTC)

A Floor Nurse or Charge Nurse in a Long-Term Care (LTC) facility (nursing home) is responsible for the day-to-day care of the residents living in the facility. CNA's and CSM's perform many of the routine cares; dressing, bathing, feeding, etc. RN's and LPN's are responsible for making sure the CNA's and CSM's carry out their duties correctly. The licensed nurses also provide specialized cares (dressing changes, injections, tube feedings, and so on) and contact the doctor when necessary.

A Charge Nurse (who may be an RN or an LPN) supervises floor staff, coordinates telephone calls, and assists the other staff members where and when needed. The Director of Nursing (DON) is available in person or by phone in case of emergency or if problems or questions arise.

In a small facility there may be only one nurse in the facility at a time; this nurse is responsible for all nursing tasks in addition to the Charge Nurse duties. In a large facility, nurses may supervise a wing, unit, or floor, with a Charge Nurse supervising the whole facility.

Pros:
* can develop a close, long-term relationship with residents and their families
* high level of independence, responsibility, and accountability
* few emergencies or critically ill residents; most residents have already determined advanced directives and do not wish to have CPR or other extraordinary measures to prolong life
* fairly predictable, although very busy, routine

Cons:
* emergency equipment may be outdated or not easily accessible
* physical stress; lots of lifting, turning, transferring residents

* nursing homes have a high level of staff turnover
* the nurse may be responsible for 50 residents or more, and the staff members caring for the residents
* CNA's are only required to complete 75 hours of education before becoming certified, and may need additional training and close supervision
* most residents are in the nursing home without possibility of discharge, and this can be depressing to care-givers
* doctors are not always responsive to a resident's needs so may not respond to a nurse's phone calls
* much paperwork and charting to meet state and federal regulations

This area may be for you if:
* you enjoy working with elderly residents and believe in making their last months or years as comfortable as possible
* you like to work with the same residents every day
* you have good supervisory skills and enjoy being in charge of CNA's and/or other nurses
* you have good organizational, prioritizing and delegating skills

This area may *not* be for you if:
* you like to give mostly direct resident/patient care
* you like to use your technical skills often
* you don't like dealing with residents and families long-term
* you find it difficult to be flexible with individual routines of the residents
* you are uncomfortable with death and dying

Other information to consider:
Doctors may or may not be responsive to Long-Term Care residents' needs. The nurse has to be a resident advocate and be willing to make many phone calls to get the residents what they need. On the other hand, a nurse working in LTC really does have the ability to make a difference in the quality of life for the residents she cares for.

There are *many* opportunities for nurses in Long Term Care; In-service Coordinator, Floor Nurse, Head Nurse, Assistant Director of Nursing, Director of Nursing, Quality Assurance, MDS +/- Coordinator, Wound Care Nurse, etc.

Skills needed:
* ability to perform a wide range of technical skills; medication administration and monitoring for adverse effects, breathing treatments, enemas, catheter insertion and care, drawing blood work, oxygen administration, dressing changes, monitoring changes in residents' conditions and applying the significance of any changes to how resident care is provided
* interpersonal skills to deal with doctors, nurses, CNA's, staff from other departments, administrators, residents, family members, state surveyors
* leadership and supervisory skills; assigning tasks appropriately, arranging tasks in order of priority, and helping staff members work together

* * * * * * * * * * * * * * * * * * * * *

Personal notes/comments:

# Home Health/Public Health

Home Health/Public Health nurses provide intermittent skilled care to patients who are homebound or find it very difficult to get to the doctor.

Home Health agencies may be privately or hospital-owned, while Public Health Agencies are state and/or federally funded.

A Home Health/Public Health patient may be of any age.

The patients are not sick enough to be admitted to a hospital or a nursing home, but do need assistance in some aspect of their daily lives. They might live alone, or family members may be unable or unwilling to provide the specialized cares or monitoring the patient needs.

A patient may be seen for a few weeks due to an acute problem such as post-surgical dressing changes, or for long- term monitoring of a chronic condition such as diabetes. Patients may be seen as frequently as once a day, or as infrequently as once a month. The frequency of the visits is ordered by the patient's doctor, and depends on the diagnosis, interventions needed, and what the patient and/or the family are able to provide.

Home Health nurses are responsible for updating the doctor about any changes or problems. Charting is vital; along with physical and mental findings the nurse must confirm the patients' homebound status and complete periodic paperwork justifying the need for continued Home Health care.

A Home Health nurse is an important resource person; s/he may refer patients to immunization, well child, and family planning clinics, Meals on Wheels, WIC, etc. The nurse also coordinates physical and/or occupational therapy, Certified Nurses Aide (to assist with ADL's), or a social worker if indicated.

Pros:
* one-to-one patient care
* satisfying to see patients quality of life improved by being at home
* rewarding to develop long-term relationships with patients and their families
* use creativity to set up individualized programs for their patients to remember to take medications, perform a dressing change correctly, or remember signs and symptoms to report to the doctor
* slower, more relaxed pace than most nursing areas, with few emergencies
* usually less physically demanding than other nursing areas
* usually work day hours during the week, with occasional evening, weekend, holiday, and on-call hours
* get to be outside of a confined environment (hospital, clinic, etc.)
* may be allowed to wear street clothes, rather than a uniform

Cons:
* a *lot* of paperwork
* pay may be less than hospital nursing
* can take a long time to establish a trusting relationship with patients; some patients will resent the fact that they need outside assistance
* patients/families may be non-compliant and/or difficult to work with
* it may take a long time to see results of nursing actions
* patients may live in poor/dirty/dangerous areas

* there is no immediate professional back-up if you have a question or problem while you are visiting a patient; for major medical emergencies, you may have to call 911
* if your patients only require monitoring, you may not get to practice your technical skills
* difficult when a patient dies, as the nurse has usually developed a long-term relationship with the patient
* may be difficult to honor the patient's wishes (remain at home) if the doctor wants the patient hospitalized for a procedure or due to illness
* little interaction with other nurses during the day
* lots of driving, chance of car trouble

This area may be for you if:
* you like working with patients with a variety of diagnoses and wide age range
* you know your way around the geographical area or are comfortable driving into unfamiliar areas, possibly in bad weather
* you like to go into patients' homes
* you like to improvise, teach, use your creativity and flexibility to help patients follow their treatment program
* you like to work long-term with patients/families
* you like one-on-one total patient care
* have good time-management skills, to get the most done for the patient at every visit
* you are comfortable making decisions independently

This area may not be for you if:
* unconventional lifestyles (unmarried couples, many pets in the home) bother you
* you are uncomfortable going into patients' homes
* you need the predictability of a set routine
* you are uncomfortable providing nursing care in untraditional ways, while still maintaining good patient care
* you would rather have support staff immediately available
* you want to use technical skills frequently
* you dislike driving, or are new to, or unfamiliar with, the geographical area
* you dislike paperwork

Other information to consider:

Home Health nurses usually don't work directly with other nurses; however, they may have patient conferences before or after visits.

The Home Health nurse must be prepared to work with patients in different ethnic groups, who may have their own customs, traditions, and beliefs.

Skills needed:
*   knowledge of and ability to perform, independently, a wide variety of technical skills; dressing changes, collecting lab specimens, setting up medications for a patient unable to do so; making sure patients take their medications correctly, monitoring weight, blood sugar, vital signs; administering blood, psychiatric monitoring and evaluation, chemotherapy, IV antibiotics, and assisting with bathing, oral care, etc.
*   assessment skills and the ability to determine signs and symptoms that merit lab work or a call to the physician, or even an Emergency Room visit
*   proficiency in interpersonal skills to deal with a variety of patients, family members, and doctors
*   ability to teach patients and their families and develop creative techniques to encourage them to take medications, perform technical tasks correctly

* * * * * * * * * * * * * * * * * * * *

Personal notes/comments:

# Hospice

To qualify for Hospice care, patients must have a terminal disease and less than six months life expectancy. Patients have chosen to die at home, with their main goal being pain relief, quality of life, and death with dignity.

Patients may be seen as frequently as once a day, or several times a week, as ordered by the patient's doctor. Hospice is similar to

Home Health nursing, as patients areseen in their homes. Home Health nurses may also visit Hospice patients.

Pros:
* usually allowed to wear street clothes rather than a uniform
* one-to-one patient care
* patients' quality of life improved by remaining at home
* slower paced than most nursing areas; advance directives and No Code orders mean the nurse does not try to *prevent* death, but provides comfort during the last months, days, and hours
* usually less physically demanding than other areas
* use creative measures to maintain patient comfort
* usually work day hours, with occasional evening, weekend, holiday, and on-call hours
* get to work outside the confined environment of a hospital, clinic, or long-term care unit
* very rewarding to be able to comfort and assist families through this extremely stressful time

Cons:
* pay may be less than that of a hospital setting
* can take a long time to establish a trusting relationship with patients and families; establishing a relationship may be hindered by the anger, sorrow, etc., the patient and family are experiencing
* patient/family may be in denial and can be non- compliant and/or difficult to work with
* patients may live in poor/dirty/dangerous areas
* no professional back-up immediately available if you need advice or assistance while visiting a patient
* difficult when a patient dies, as the nurse has developed a close relationship with the patient and family
* may not use technical skills on a daily basis
* no patients get "better"
* can be difficult to provide patient comfort if the doctor is not receptive to increasing pain medication or other comfort measures
* little interaction with other nurses during the day
* this area can become depressing for the nurse
* lots of driving; potential for adverse weather conditions or car trouble

This area may be for you if:
* you don't mind working with patients who have a terminal diagnosis
* you know your way around the geographical area or are comfortable driving into unfamiliar areas, possibly in bad weather
* you like to go into patients' homes
* you like to improvise, teach, use your creativity and flexibility to help patients be as comfortable as possible
* you enjoy working long-term with patients/families
* you like one-on-one total patient care
* have good time-management skills, to get the most done for the patient at every visit
* you can provide emotional support for patients and family members

This area may not be for you if:
* you are not comfortable knowing your patients have a terminal diagnosis
* you are not comfortable talking about death and dying
* you need to see patients get well
* unconventional lifestyles (unmarried couples, many pets in the home) bother you
* you are uncomfortable going into patients' homes
* you need the predictability of set routines
* you are uncomfortable providing nursing care in untraditional ways, while still maintaining good patient care
* you would rather have support staff immediately available
* you want to use technical skills frequently
* you dislike driving, or are new to, or unfamiliar with, the geographical area

Other information to consider:
Hospice nurses develop very close relationships with patients and their families. They may attend a patient's funeral, and keep in touch with the family for several months after the patient dies.

Skills needed:
* knowledge of, and ability to perform, independently, a wide variety of technical skills; dressing changes, collecting lab specimens, setting up medications for a patient unable to do so; making sure patients take their medications correctly,

monitoring weight, blood sugar, vital signs; administering blood, psychiatric monitoring and evaluation, chemotherapy, IV antibiotics, and assisting with bathing, oral care, and comfort measures
* assessment skills and the ability to determine signs and symptoms that merit lab work or a call to the physician
* proficiency in interpersonal skills to deal with a variety of patients, family members, and doctors
* interpersonal skills to listen to patients and family members share feelings related to life, death, and dying
* ability to teach patients and their families and develop creative techniques to encourage them to take medications, perform technical tasks correctly, and comfort the dying patient

* * * * * * * * * * * * * * * * * * * *

Personal notes/comments:

# Clinic/Doctor's Office

Family practice clinic or office nurses see a wide variety of patients-OB, pediatric, cardiac, orthopedic, geriatric, etc. A nurse who prefers more specialized work may choose a more specialized clinic; high-risk pregnancies, or an eye clinic, for example.

The clinic nurse prepares patients to be seen by the doctor, performs basic tests, and carries out any doctor's orders. S/he may spend much of the day on the phone answering questions and giving advice to patients. As the nurse becomes familiar with the physician's management of routine problems, s/he can ask pertinent questions, suggest at-home remedies, and ask the patient to come to the clinic if s/he knows the physician would prefer to see the patient.

Pros:
* day hours and possible Saturdays—no major holidays
* opportunity to learn about many different illnesses and conditions

97

* pleasant, clean environment
* busy pace, but few crisis situations
* develop long-term relationships with patients

Cons:
* pay may not be comparable to that of hospitals
* may not use technical skills on a daily basis
* may miss occasional daytime activities of children in school

This area may be for you if:
* you do not care for working in a hospital or nursing home
* you enjoy working closely with doctors, patients, and families
* you enjoy gathering information and teaching, both over the phone and in person

This area may *not* be for you if:
* you enjoy crisis situations
* you prefer to utilize more specialized technical skills
* you do not enjoy teaching patients and their families

Other information to consider:
If you have children in school, you may be able to schedule your hours so you are home when they leave for and/or arrive home after school. Depending on the size of the office, it may be fairly easy, or difficult, to arrange for time off for school or other family events. If this is a major factor in your decision to apply at a clinic, discuss the policy for time off before accepting a job at a clinic.

Skills needed:
* technical skills; good history-taking and assessment skills; the ability to ask detailed questions and gather pertinent information about the patient's complaint(s)
* technical skills; blood draws, urinalysis, pulmonary function tests, X-Rays, and other lab tests done in the office; injections, immunizations
* good interpersonal skills when working with patients in person and on the telephone

* * * * * * * * * * * * * * * * * * * *

Personal notes/comments:

# Occupational Health/Industrial

An Occupational Health Nurse or Industrial Nurse provides first-aid, health education and screenings, and various types of safety and educational training in an industrial setting (packing plant, factory, etc.). S/he provides emergency first aid when needed, in the case of an injury, accident, chemical spill, or other emergency. The nurse may be responsible for the Hearing Conservation Program and/or other OSHA (Occupational Safety and Health Administration) regulations.

Pros:
* day hours, weekends and holidays off
* good pay and benefits
* few emergencies or crisis situations

Cons:
* few, if any, other health care professionals in the setting
* lack of exposure to procedures and basic nursing skills
* lots of paperwork required to comply with regulations

This area may be for you if:
* you prefer day hours
* you enjoy teaching
* you like a relaxed pace of working

This area may *not* be for you if:
* you don't enjoy paperwork
* you like to use technical nursing skills on a daily basis

Other information to consider:
Jobs in this area are limited. Employees may be reluctant to attend required classes or follow safety routines which they see as unnecessary.

Skills needed:
*   basic first-aid and nursing skills
*   good teaching skills regarding safety issues
*   good interpersonal skills for working with employees who may be non-compliant in following regulations

* * * * * * * * * * * * * * * * * * * *

Personal notes/comments:

# Hemodialysis—Chronic

Patients with chronic kidney failure require hemodialysis in an out-patient hemodialysis center. The pace is fairly relaxed in a dialysis center. Patients may be dialyzed several times a week, for several hours at a time. Most patients require dialysis until transplant is possible or death occurs.

Acute dialysis is discussed on page 87.

Pros:
*   excellent learning opportunity for the nurse to gain specialized skills
*   relaxed pace of work
*   opportunity to develop a long-term relationship with patients

Cons:
*   long hours (clinics may be open 5 AM - 7 PM), may have "on-call" hours
*   dealing with chronic patients who may be non-compliant and not follow dietary and medical regime
*   patients may have many medical problems
*   routine may become boring

This area may be for you if:
*   you enjoy working with patients long-term
*   you have excellent IV skills and enjoy using them

* you enjoy interpreting lab values and adjusting treatment accordingly
* enjoy working at a more relaxed pace

This area may *not* be for you if:
* you do not enjoy working with patients long-term
* you have trouble accepting that treatment and teaching may improve patient status but that patients do not "get better"

Other information to consider:
    Chronic hemodialysis patients may be very non-compliant. This can be frustrating to the nurse who has taken a lot of time to teach the patient, only to find s/he is not following instructions.
    Many smaller communities (less than 10,000 people) are offering hemodialysis clinics, so chronic patients do not have to travel as far for dialysis.

Skills needed:
* excellent assessment skills: of lab results, cardiac and respiratory status, fluid and electrolyte balance
* technical skills: IV, mechanical (dialysis machines), and assessment, interpretation of lab results and interventions as necessary
* interpersonal skills, especially with long-term patients who may be non-compliant, depressed, etc.
* teaching patients about the process of dialysis, and dietary restrictions

* * * * * * * * * * * * * * * * * *

Personal notes/comments:

# Traveling

A traveling nurse is employed by an agency, which sends her to hospitals or other health-care facilities requiring temporary additional staffing, usually due to seasonal needs. For example, facilities in warm climates need more nurses during the winter, when people travel to these climates.

A nurse signs on with a traveling agency, which assigns her to a geographical area and nursing area in which she is interested in working. The traveling nurse usually interviews, via phone, with the person who will be supervising her in the facility in which she will be working. Assignments generally last from four to twenty-six weeks, depending on the needs of the facility. A nurse from the agency assists the traveling nurse in relocating (usually in agency-sponsored housing), obtaining licensure, and making sure the assignment goes smoothly. A nurse may take a permanent assignment if she wants to relocate permanently, if that facility has a position open. Positions in all specialty areas are needed, in all areas of the United States.

Pros:
* opportunity to see different areas of the United States and meet many new people
* opportunity to use specialty nursing skills in various facilities
* very good pay and benefits offered
* can take time off between job assignments

Cons:
* many changes, may be difficult to get used to different facilities
* some agencies may not provide benefits promised; job nurse was hired for may be unavailable when the nurse gets there
* permanent staff nurses may be unwilling to help the traveling nurse become oriented with the area

This area may be for you if:
* you are flexible, quick to adapt, and thrive on change
* you are a team player
* you are well organized, detail oriented

This area may *not* be for you if:
* you are comfortable where you are

* you cannot relocate easily
* you do not like change

Other information about this area:
If you would like to be a traveling nurse, call several of the agencies advertised in nursing magazines. Compare pay and benefits, and talk with a nurse who has worked with that company.

One year of experience in the area in which you will be working, is required. You are required to be eligible for licensure in the state in which you will be working.

Skills needed:
* technical skills in the area in which you will be working (see specific areas in the other chapters of this section)
* interpersonal skills to work with nurses and doctors, as well as patients
* flexibility, adaptability, the ability to deal with change and quickly learn different routines

* * * * * * * * * * * * * * * * * * * *

Personal notes/comments:

# Prison

A prison nurse may work in a men's or women's prison, or in a prison hospital. A prison nurse may be a primary nurse for a number of patients with chronic problems such as asthma or diabetes, and see these patients on a regular basis.

The prison nurse has a very high level of independence—in diagnosing problems, initiating the treatment plan (from standing orders given by physicians), and making decisions regarding medical interventions. The prison nurse may have access to only very basic diagnostic tools—blood pressure cuff, thermometer, stethoscope—and have to use his or her assessment skills, knowledge, and "gut instincts" to determine whether or not the prisoner's complaint is serious and legitimate.

The prison nurse must deal with routine complaints such as sore throats and headaches, as well as serious injuries like blunt trauma, knife wounds, overdoses, and suicide attempts.

Pros:
* very high level of independence

Cons:
* physical, verbal, and sexual harassment and abuse from prisoners
* few "warm fuzzies" from patients
* have to deal with complaints of prisoners, as well as pressures from management to keep the prisoners happy while keeping costs down
* a large amount of charting and paperwork

This area may be for you if:
* you are comfortable working independently (although there may be other nurses on the premises and a physician on call)
* you are authoritative and able to deal with abuse
* you are able to work with patients who have little or no formal education, or who place little value on life
* the idea of working with prisoners—who may be violent—does not bother you
* you are able to deal with emergencies such as stabbings, drug overdoses, and hangings

This area may *not* be for you if:
* you are not confident of your nursing judgement and nursing skills
* you are not comfortable acting independently
* you need a lot of positive feedback in order to feel job satisfaction

Other information to consider:
Most prison nurses must be RN's and have at least one year of experience; trauma and/or ER experience is especially helpful. Pay and benefits may or may not be comparable to other nursing jobs in the geographical area. Prison nursing is a *very* challenging area of nursing!

Skills needed:
* excellent assessment skills, using limited diagnostic tools
* assessment and intervention skills to deal with stabbings, blunt trauma, etc.
* excellent interpersonal skills to deal with violent, abusive, manipulative patients
* wide range of nursing skills (IV's, chest tubes, medication administration, dressing changes) if working in a prison hospital (fewer nursing skills are used in a general prison as sick or severely injured patients are transferred to a local hospital or prison hospital)

* * * * * * * * * * * * * * * * * * * * *

Personal notes/comments:

# Private Duty

Private duty nurses may care for patients in their home, Long Term Care (LTC) facility, or in the hospital. A private duty patient may range in age from newborn to geriatric, and have diagnoses including Cerebral Palsy, stroke, paralysis, dementia, or any other condition requiring skilled care.

Hospital or LTC patients usually need private duty nurses for reasons such as agitation or extreme confusion, necessitating one-to-one supervision and nursing care. Family members may feel more comfortable with the one-to-one attention a private duty nurse provides, even if this is not medically necessary.

Private duty patients in the home are usually in stable condition. The private duty nurse may provide relief for family members who care for these patients needing constant monitoring, or the nurse may be needed because family members are unable or unwilling to care for the patient. S/he or he may also provide any skilled care needed.

(See Home Health for more information about caring for a patient in his or her home)

Pros:
* just one patient to care for!
* chance to develop a close relationship with the patient
* you usually get to choose the days and shifts you work, and may not have to work full eight hour shifts, allowing you to meet *your* needs and the needs of your family
* patients are usually medically stable, although their condition may change at any time
* pay is comparable to, or higher than, hospital pay
* chance to feel good about your job, seeing the difference you can make in a patient's quality of life

Cons:
* some nurses find that working with just one patient is less stimulating or challenging
* no other nurses or doctors, emergency medications, crash cart, etc. immediately available in the case of an emergency
* scheduled shifts will be cancelled if the patient goes into the hospital, and with some patients this happens very frequently and with little advance notice
* death of a patient can be hard to take after spending time together

This area may be for you if:
* you like to work with patients and their families
* you can provide good patient care while being flexible with your routine, so patient and family needs can be met
* you enjoy working with just one patient
* you like to work independently

This area may *not* be for you if:
* you like to work with more than one patient at a time
* you are uncomfortable working in a home, without immediate medical back-up available
* you prefer the excitement of working in a hospital
* you need to work a guaranteed number of hours each week

Other information to consider:
The private duty patient and his or her family are usually very knowledgeable about the patient's condition, medications, treatments, etc.

You may find private duty assignments through your local hospital, or by applying with a private duty agency. The employer will offer you assignments in your geographical and nursing specialty area. You may arrange your own schedule based on the needs of the patients and family. You may decide to work mainly with one family, or see a different patient each day of the week, depending on the number of patients in your geographical area.

Skills needed:
* technical skills required vary according to patient needs and may include; respiratory treatments, tube feedings IV fluids or medications; the patient may be on a ventilator, using oxygen, or monitored by an oximeter or apnea monitor
* good interpersonal skills to work with a patient and his or her family

* * * * * * * * * * * * * * * * * * * * *

Personal notes/comments:

# School

The school nurse's function is to promote a healthy environment to maximize the student's potential to learn. For the student, this includes assessing and removing health- related barriers by such means as health and wellness counselling, guidance, home visits, and referrals to community agencies like AlAteen, social services, etc.

The school nurse maintains student health records. The school nurse serves as a resource person for other teachers, providing inservice programs, safety management, and basic first aid training. The school nurse acts as a liaison person between the students, the school, and the community.

Pros:
* Monday through Friday, day hours, no weekends, holidays, or summers!
* work independently
* can increase income by working during the summer

Cons:
* no professional backup immediately available in case of emergency
* wages may not be competitive with health care facilities
* can be discouraging to see kids engaging in unsafe health practices

This area may be for you if:
* you like to work with kids
* you enjoy teaching and counselling
* you are comfortable talking about subjects like drugs, sex, AIDS, teen-age pregnancy, abuse (by parents or boy or girl-friends)
* you have kids in school, as you will be off when they are

This area may *not* be for you if:
* you are disturbed by difficult student/family situations
* you do not like working with kids
* you need a competitive wage

Other information about this area:
A school nurse must be prepared to deal with students in a tremendous variety of situations; abuse, pregnancy, drug use, depression, death in the family, etc., etc. The nurse must be able to be supportive and suggest the options the student may have, in any of these situations.

Skills needed:
* basic assessment and technical skills when performing health screenings or assessing a sick student
* basic first aid knowledge to care for injured students
* superior interpersonal skills to deal with a wide variety of student situations

* * * * * * * * * * * * * * * * * * * *

# Camp

A camp nurse provides routine and emergency care for children attending camp. Campers may spend only day time hours at camp (day camp) or days and nights (sleep-away camp). Camp sessions may last from two weeks to several months.

The camp nurse must obtain consent forms from parents. The signed consents allow the nurse to administer routine medications (allergy shots, allergy medications, over-the- counter cold and pain relievers, etc.), and treat the camper for routine and emergency problems.

The nurse must be prepared to deal with emergencies related to camp activities—sunburn, heat stroke, archery accidents, horse-riding accidents, drowning, broken bones, snake bites—although the main complaint of campers is homesickness.

Camps may be for children with spina bifida, diabetes, or other special needs. The nurse working at a specialized camp must be familiar with these conditions and potential problems that may arise.

The camp nurse has a unique opportunity to teach kids about CPR, the Heimlich Maneuver, safety, and health-care careers—when outdoor activities are cancelled due to rain. Several nurses may be employed by a camp, or the nurse maybe the only health-care professional available.

Pros:
*   nurse's family may be able to attend camp free or at reduced rates
*   the nurse may take part in recreational activities offered by the camp; crafts, swimming, archery, hiking, etc.
*   relaxed pace; few, if any, emergencies
*   time to catch up on reading
*   minimal charting!
*   short-term; sessions generally last from two weeks to several months

* room and board provided; travel allowance and licensure in state where camp takes place may be provided
* pay generally good, considering room and board provided

Cons:
* may be difficult to get time off from regular job to work at a camp
* "on-call" at all hours except for days off
* there might not be any other nurses or doctors available to consult or assist if there is an emergency
* may or may not have private accommodations; may have to share bathroom/shower facilities
* can be somewhat boring; may not utilize nursing skills
* away from family if they do not attend camp

This area may be for you if:
* you enjoy spending time in the country
* you like being with kids and can communicate with them; many times physical complaints are relieved by a sympathetic listener.
* you are outgoing and enjoy participating in a variety of camp activities.
* you are comfortable being independent
* you are confident about your ability to act appropriately in emergency situations

This area may *not* be for you if:
* you can't get time off to work at a camp
* you like to use technical nursing skills daily
* you do not like to be the only health-care professional available
* you don't like being away from home; you will miss take-out food, attending movies, shopping at the mall
* you don't have the patience to talk to kids

Other information to consider:
Camp nurse opportunities can be found in the "help wanted" section of nursing magazines.
Camp nurses have a unique opportunity to influence young people by educating them about basic health issues and career opportunities in health care.

Camp nursing is a great change of pace for a nurse who is burned out.

A camp nurse needs to be licensed in the state s/he will be working in; the camp may or may not pay for the license.

Skills needed:
* basic assessment skills; the ability to treat routine problems and emergencies
* interpersonal skills for gaining the confidence of parents and campers; interacting with kids and other camp employees

* * * * * * * * * * * * * * * * * * * *

Personal notes/comments:

# Flight

A flight nurse cares for a critically ill or injured patient who requires rapid transport, via specially equipped helicopters, to a hospital equipped to care for the patient.
The helicopter may pick up a patient at the site of an accident or at the transferring hospital.

Helicopters may be staffed with teams consisting of nurse/paramedic, nurse/nurse, or nurse/physician. Nurses follow program protocols and standing orders when maintaining airway management and administering treatments and medications.

Problems unique to flight nursing include; difficulty maintaining oxygen saturation while in the low oxygen altitude, and maintaining the flow of IV's—many times a pump is required.

Pros:
* work with "cutting edge" technology and equipment
* get to fly!
* very high level of independence; if there are two patients on-scene, the nurse works completely independently on one of the patients
* very rapid-paced

Cons:
*   limited space in the helicopter (although fully equipped with monitoring equipment)
*   noisy in the helicopter, making it difficult to communicate with the patient and other nurse/paramedic/physician
*   highly visible to the public, who criticize/comment on performance of flight nurses

This area may be for you if:
*   you enjoy a very fast-paced job
*   you are able to make quick decisions independently
*   you are assertive, confident, and have a strong personality
*   you enjoy working in a "high-tech" environment

This area may *not* be for you if:
*   you don't like stress
*   you are afraid of flying or get air-sick!!
*   you do not like to make decisions independently or take a long time to make decision
*   you would rather work in a more predictable area

Other information to consider:
A flight nurse must meet physical requirements which include; lifting a patient in and out of the helicopter, moving around in the helicopter, etc. Some programs may have weight and height and other fitness regulations.

A flight nurse must have four to five years of ICU and/or ER experience. ACLS, PALS, BTLS, and other trauma certification may be required as a prerequisite, or as part of training. Some programs require that the nurse also be a paramedic. During flight nurse training, the nurse will learn about aviation, as well as nursing cares while in flight.

Due to extensive training required, a nurse who wishes to become a flight nurse should carefully consider this decision.

Skills necessary:
*   advanced technical skills: airway management, starting and maintaining IV's, assessing the patient's condition and acting according to protocol
*   ability to work with advanced equipment—ventilators, IV pumps, defibrillators, etc.

* knowledge of, and ability to work around, difficulties encountered when flying
* interpersonal skills to quickly establish a relationship with the patient and tactfully deal with bystanders
* willingness to undergo lengthy and strenuous training

* * * * * * * * * * * * * * * * * * * *

Personal notes/comments:

# Insurance Exams

Performing insurance exams involves going to clients' homes and places of employment to conduct a basic physical examination, as requested by the insurance company which is writing a policy on that individual.

Pros:
* flexible hours (can usually schedule exams when it fits *your* schedule)
* very short-term, one time, one-to-one contact with clients
* use and maintain basic nursing skills
* no critical or emergency situations
* may wear casual clothes

Cons:
* sometimes hard to schedule appointments to fit into both your schedule and your client's
* may have to travel to the client's home and may or may not be reimbursed for travel time and/or mileage
* may have to take specimens (UA, blood samples) to the post office to mail them
* hours are not consistent

This area may be for you if:
* you enjoy working one-to-one with people for a very short time

113

* you don't mind traveling
* your work/personal schedule is flexible
* you enjoy working with well "patients"

This area may *not* be for you if:
* you need a steady income, as you only do exams (and get paid) when the insurance company sells policies
* you prefer to work with patients for a longer period of time
* you like to use advanced nursing skills

Other information to consider:
See the sections "Home Health" and "Hospice" for other information on working with clients in their homes.

Skills needed:
* basic technical skills; obtaining vital signs, height, weight, blood and urine specimens, family history
* interpersonal skills to quickly establish a trusting relationship with clients
* basic teaching skills to explain procedures such as checking blood pressure, collection of blood and urine specimens, etc.

* * * * * * * * * * * * * * * * * * * *

Personal notes/comments:

# Parish

Parish nursing began in 1984. Parish nurses work to make health care more accessible to members of their congregation. Parish nursing is interdemoninational. A parish nurse has the opportunity to assist in the wholistic care of the patient, including spiritual needs, which are often overlooked or forgotten.

A parish nurse does not provide direct patient care, but rather provides counseling, education, and spiritual and emotional support.

A parish nurse, unlike nurses in more traditional roles, is encouraged to promote spiritual wellness through Bible study, prayer, and spiritual discussion with her patients.

Parish nurses may visit patients in the hospital, nursing home, or in their home. S/he may keep regular "office hours" at a church or synagogue.

Pros:
*   develop very close relationships with patients
*   get to know members of the congregation
*   work one-to-one with patients
*   become familiar with community services
*   very satisfying to help patients solve problems and assist them in getting necessary medical care
*   get to share the spiritual side of yourself
*   little or no charting!

Cons:
*   pay (most parish nurses volunteer their time; they may receive money for gas, educational supplies, and so on)

This area may be for you if:
*   you are comfortable with your spirituality, sharing your beliefs, and praying with others
*   you enjoy listening to your patients
*   you enjoy problem solving and organizing volunteers
*   you are comfortable working one-to-one with patients in their homes (see Home Health for more information)
*   you would rather provide more emotional and spiritual support than physical care
*   you enjoy teaching

This area may not be for you if:
*   you are not comfortable with your own spirituality
*   you need a steady income
*   you would rather provide physical cares

Other information about this area:
A parish nurse may be employed by his or her congregation, or by a church-affiliated hospital. Most parish nurses volunteer their time, although some are paid. Liability insurance is a must; even though parish nurses do not provide physical cares, they do give ad-

vice and suggest interventions. Most parish nurses create their own jobs by approaching the congregation with a proposal outlining the need for a parish nurse program and how it can be implemented. For more information, contact: The National Parish Nurse Resource Center at 1-800-556-5368; or The Health Ministries Association at 1-800-852-5613.

Skills needed:
*    the ability to see needs for teaching, volunteers, referral to community services, support groups, and fill these needs
*    basic knowledge of anatomy and physiology, medications, and illness prevention, and the ability and willingness to teach laypeople about these areas
*    ability to teach people with various education levels
*    interpersonal skills for dealing with families and individuals in times of crisis

* * * * * * * * * * * * * * * * * * * *

Personal notes/comments:

# Blood Mobile

A nurse working with the Red Cross Blood Mobile collects blood from volunteer donors and transports the blood to hospitals or storage centers. Collection may be done in a permanent building designed for blood donation, or equipment may be transferred to a temporary site (city hall, gymnasium, etc.).

The nurse working for the Blood Mobile does a Health History Assessment on potential donors (who must meet certain health and health history guidelines). The nurse then collects the blood and transports it, adhering to strict standards which assure the blood remains pure.

Pros:
*    work with healthy people
*    very good benefits—uniforms, licensure, etc.

* no lifting of, or transferring patients
* use basic assessment and technical skills daily

Cons:
* long hours
* must work within very strict and regimented guidelines

This area may be for you if:
* you can work long hours
* you can work according to strict standards
* you like to travel
* you are able to immediately establish a trusting relationship with blood donors

This area may not be for you if:
* you want to use specialized nursing skills daily
* you don't like to travel
* you like to use creativity in your work

Other information to consider:
The Red Cross provides a six-week orientation for new employees. During this time, nurses learn about policies and procedures, and observe. They are closely monitored in all aspects of compliance to policies regarding the collection, storage, and safekeeping of blood products.

Skills needed:
* basic history taking, assessment, and technical skills (vital signs, finger stick for blood sample)
* ability to follow strict standards
* interpersonal skills to deal with various personalities of donors and co-workers

* * * * * * * * * * * * * * * * * * * * *

Personal notes/comments:

# Indirect Patient Care Areas
## *In-Hospital*

## Supervisory Positions

### TEAM LEADER

In team nursing, an RN Team Leader may be responsible for several other RN's or LPN's as well as their patients. S/he may or may not be assigned patients. The Team Leader RN supervises other nurses, acts as a resource person, and does treatments and procedures that other personnel are not licensed or qualified to do; IV's for example. The Team Leader may make calls to the lab, pharmacy, doctors, etc., for the other nurses on the team. The Team Leader is responsible, in most cases, for the care given by the other nurses on the team. Responsibilities may vary according to facility policy.

Pros:
* usually do not perform routine tasks such as bathing, medication administration
* perform, or assist with, challenging procedures

Cons:
* may be in charge of many patients, incompetent nurses, etc.

A Team Leader position may be for you if:
* you don't mind making phone calls
* you are comfortable supervising others
* you are willing and able to teach other nurses about medications, treatments, and other aspects of patient care
* you have good organizational and assessment skills and can set priorities and help other nurses set priorities
* you do not enjoy routine "hands on" nursing

A Team Leader position may *not* be for you if:
* you do not like to be in charge of other nurses
* you prefer "hands on" care and close contact with patients

* you are a new graduate, as you must be proficient at—and comfortable with—all aspects of patient care and have leadership skills that come with experience

Other information to consider:

A Team Leader must be proficient in all aspects of patient care. S/he must be comfortable assigning tasks and teaching other nurses. As you become acquainted with your team members' abilities, Team Leading will be easier as you'll become familiar with team members strengths and weaknesses.

Skills needed:
* assessment skills to monitor patients of the nurses she is supervising
* technical skills to assist and teach other nurses when necessary
* interpersonal skills to work with and direct nurses and other hospital personnel; patients, families, and doctors, and mediate and diffuse any conflicts
* supervisory skills to assign patients to nurses appropriately, supervise care provided

* * * * * * * * * * * * * * * * * * * * *

Personal notes/comments:

## CHARGE NURSE

For the purpose of this book, a Charge Nurse is in charge of a floor, unit, or facility for a shift; s/he may or may not be permanently assigned as a Charge Nurse. Check facility policy for specific Charge Nurse job description. The Charge Nurse is responsible for overseeing patient care and is usually not assigned to care for specific patients. S/he assists when necessary: inserting a difficult IV, coordinating patient transfers, admissions, or dismissals, making telephone calls, etc. The Charge Nurse also diffuses conflicts between staff members, staff and patients, patients and doctors, etc.

Pros:
* "in charge"
* little charting, unless performing direct patient care
* usually paid a Charge Nurse differential

Cons:
* responsible for any and all aspects of patient care provided during the shift s/he is in charge
* must deal with difficult technical and interpersonal situations
* may have to deal with difficult and/or less competent nurses and other personnel

A Charge Nurse Position may be for you if:
* you are well organized, confident, and can set priorities
* you can perform appropriately in crisis situations
* you would rather coordinate care than perform hands-on patient care
* you are comfortable with, and able to perform, difficult technical skills
* you like to teach
* your goal is a management position

A Charge Nurse position may *not* be for you if:
* you would rather be responsible for hands-on, total patient care
* you don't like being in charge
* you are uncomfortable supervising nurses and handling conflicts

Other information to consider:
If you are interested in a management position, being a Charge Nurse is a great place to start. Charge Nurses are needed on all shifts, and you can get a taste of what management involves without the full-time commitment of a Head Nurse or D.O.N. position.

Skills needed:
* knowledge of, and ability to perform, technical skills in difficult situations
* excellent interpersonal skills; the ability to resolve conflicts between staff members, staff and patients, etc.
* leadership skills to assure good patient care is provided
* confidence in yourself and your decisions

120

Personal notes/comments:

## HEAD NURSE

The Head Nurse of each floor or unit assumes 24 hour/7 day a week responsibility for the patient care provided in that specific on which s/he is Head Nurse. Depending on facility policy, and nursing availability, the education and experience requirements for a Head Nurse may vary; it is standard practice that a Head Nurse be an RN with at least some experience in the area in which s/he is Head Nurse.

The Head Nurse is responsible for staffing the area, around the clock, to provide good, safe, patient care. Depending on facility policy, patient census, and staffing, the Head Nurse is usually not required to provide direct patient care. S/he is used as a resource person and is available to assist with a difficult patient or procedure or in case of emergency (code situation). The Head Nurse must make sure the staff is sufficiently qualified, educated, and trained, to provide an acceptable standard of care. S/he is also responsible for personnel management—evaluations, counseling, etc.

Pros:
*   usually a Monday through Friday day position; but on call 24 hours a day/7 days a week
*   self-satisfaction at meeting a professional goal of supervising
*   helping other nurses reach professional goals
*   new challenges every day
*   seeing changes you implement having a positive effect on patient care

Cons:
*   never leave your job at work; "on-call" 24 hours a day/7 days a week
*   work much more than 40 hours per week
*   infrequent use of technical nursing skills

*    have to be the "bad guy" when disciplining, etc.
*    may have to work on the floor if no one else is available

A Head Nurse position may be for you if:
*    your goal is a supervisory position
*    you are willing to devote a tremendous amount of time to your job
*    you are highly motivated and willing to stay abreast of changes related to nursing
*    your self-esteem does not depend on being liked by everyone on the floor as none of your decisions will be liked by everyone

A Head Nurse position is not for you if:
*    you do not have strong family support
*    you are uncomfortable with the tasks of counseling, reprimands, terminations, etc.
*    you don't have a strong survival instinct

Other information to consider:
A Head Nurse must constantly show his or her staff willingness and ability to function effectively in all roles.

*"You never totally leave your job at work—it's like a child, always requiring a certain amount of nurturing and follow-up."*
Teressa Williams, RN

Skills needed:
*    knowledge of, and ability to, perform technical skills in difficult situations
*    interpersonal skills to deal with conflicts between staff, doctors, patients, families, or all of the above!
*    able to gain the support and cooperation of staff in implementing new procedures, providing good, safe, patient care
*    interpersonal skills, basic management skills, and willingness to deal with personnel issues; counseling, personality conflicts, etc.
*    ability to be a patient *and* nurse advocate

* * * * * * * * * * * * * * * * * * * * *

Personal notes/comments:

# Management Positions

*"One piece of advice to new graduates—don't be too anxious to take on a job and responsibilities for which you have no or little experience . . . this is particularly true in the area of administration."* Rose Waddell, RN

## DIRECTOR OF NURSING—HOSPITAL

A hospital Director of Nursing (DON) is responsible for making sure quality nursing care is provided in all areas of nursing in the facility in which s/he works.

The DON is ultimately responsible for recruiting, hiring, training, evaluating, and providing leadership and guidance to nursing personnel, managing patient care, developing and monitoring departmental budgets, as well as attending numerous meetings and workshops.

The DON continually works to *improve* nursing care provided, assures standards of nursing care and practice are met, develops and follows policies and procedures for nursing care, and assures compliance with JCAHO, Department of Health, Medicare, and other regulatory agencies. S/he must maintain effective working relationships with physicians, other health care professionals, and patients and their family members.

A DON must be available 24 hours a day for consultation, and in small facilities, to assist in emergency situations that require additional RN assistance—a patient with an acute MI, for example. A DON in a small facility may also be on-call to assist in Labor and Delivery and for any unexpected surgeries.

The DON is in a position that is accessible to the public; s/he must present a positive image of the hospital.

Pros:
* satisfying to be "in charge" and have a say in policies, procedures, how the hospital is run, etc.
* day shift, Monday through Friday hours except in case of emergencies
* less physical work than general floor nursing

Cons:
* hours worked are usually much greater than 40 per week
* on-call 24 hours a day in case of emergencies, questions, or concerns
* ultimately responsible for all patient care provided
* usually very little direct patient contact
* in a small facility, the DON may have to work on the floor if staffing is short
* may be difficult to deal with disciplinary, employee, and facility problems

A DON position may be for you if:
* you work well with people
* you are comfortable making decisions, knowing that they may not be popular decisions
* you have excellent delegation skills
* have general knowledge of all areas of nursing
* like doing *lots* of paperwork
* able to work with staff from different departments and work together to make decisions
* able to work through difficult situations which may involve doctors, nurses, other hospital personnel, patients, families, or all of the above!

A DON position may *not* be for you if:
* you are uncomfortable making managerial decisions
* you would rather do "hands-on" nursing
* don't like paperwork

Other information to consider:
State and federal regulations require a DON to be a full-time employee.

The DON may not get a lot of positive feedback; s/he must be able to take *personal* satisfaction in work well done.

Skills needed:
* knowledge of and ability to perform technical nursing skills
* interpersonal skills for dealing with conflicts among and between nurses, doctors, other hospital personnel, patients, families
* interpersonal skills for working with staff members from different departments, administration, etc.

* leadership/supervisory skills necessary to assure good patient care
* knowledge of to whom certain tasks can be delegated
* leadership/supervisory skills necessary to deal with staff members in various situations
* management skills when dealing with staff members, regulations, projects, etc.

\* \* \* \* \* \* \* \* \* \* \* \* \* \* \* \* \* \* \* \*

Personal notes/comments:

## ASSISTANT DIRECTOR OF NURSING— HOSPITAL OR LONG-TERM CARE

The job description for an Assistant Director of Nursing (ADON) may be very similar to a Director of Nursing's (DON's). The ADON works with the DON and is responsible for tasks delegated by the DON, which may include Infection Control, monitoring lab results, planning the schedule, and so on. (see Director of Nursing—Long-Term Care and Hospital for responsibilities of the DON))

Pros:
* day hours, Monday through Friday
* may not have to work full-time (the DON is required to work full-time)
* management position without the full responsibility the DON carries

Cons:
* may have to check with the DON before making decisions
* could be assigned undesirable tasks the DON does not want to do
* job description can change frequently

An ADON position may be for you if:
* you can be loyal to the DON, and publicly stand behind her decisions
* you work well with other managers
* you want to try a management position without the responsibility of a DON position

An ADON position may *not* be for you if:
* you want to make independent decisions
* you do not want to share management responsibilities

Other information to consider:

The relationship between the DON and ADON is of the utmost importance in forming a productive working environment. If responsibilities are not *clearly* defined, or either person does not want to work with the other, the working relationship may be difficult; one person taking (or being assigned) the undesirable tasks, and/or some important tasks not getting done at all! Communication is vital.

The ADON may not have to work a 40 hour week.

* * * * * * * * * * * * * * * * * * * *

Personal notes/comments:

## HOUSE SUPERVISOR

A House Supervisor is delegated to oversee an entire facility, from housekeeping to radiology to nursing. In many facilities, a House Supervisor is present during every shift. The House Supervisor is responsible for making sure facility policy is followed throughout the establishment, and the standard of care is maintained. The House Supervisor serves as a resource person and consults on patient care problems, delegates, and problem solves as necessary. The House Supervisor must work with other Head Nurses and/or Charge Nurses, and department heads in making sure every aspect of patient care runs smoothly.

126

Pros:
  * feeling of accomplishment to be "in charge"
  * exposed to all areas of patient care
  * rewarding to know you are looked upon as a resource person
  * satisfying to be able to see the "big picture" regarding patient care
  * get to "visit" all areas of the facility

Cons:
  * not everyone likes every decision you make
  * people may not be happy to see you—unless they need something
  * may have to find staff when staffing is short
  * have to make unpopular decisions, like pulling and floating staff
  * must spend a lot of time on the phone
  * can be stressful to work with doctors; for example, when a doctor wants his patient in ICU, no bed is available, yet he demands that you get a bed
  * may have long hours, weekends, holidays
  * pay differential may not make up for increased responsibilities
  * may have to make some administrative decisions, and handle problems administration usually handles, on weekends or hours administration is not available
  * little or no direct patient contact

A House Supervisor position may be for you if:
  * you have good leadership skills
  * you do not mind making unpopular or difficult decisions
  * you have excellent communication skills, and enjoy using them in difficult situations
  * you have excellent problem-solving skills

A House Supervisor position may not be for you if:
  * you cannot think "on your feet" and make difficult decisions
  * you prefer direct patient care
  * you do not like the responsibility
  * you do not have the desire, or ability, to work with people from all departments of the facility

Other information about this area:

The House Supervisor must have confidence in his or herself, abilities, and decisions. The House Supervisor may be confronted with very touchy situations; for example, a father wanting to see his baby but the unwed mother not wanting him to have any contact with the baby. A House Supervisor must be prepared to deal with any situation!

Skills needed:
* broad base of knowledge of technical skills used in every area of the facility
* interpersonal skills for dealing with staff issues, patients, doctors, nurses, families; the difficult cases will be brought to the House Supervisor!
* knowledge of policies and procedures, to assure quality patient care takes place while s/he is on duty
* organizational skills to assess staffing needs; interpersonal skills to make unpopular decisions to assure staffing needs are met
* leadership and management skills to assure all departments are working together, according to facility policy, to assure good patient care

* * * * * * * * * * * * * * * * * * * *

Personal notes/comments:

# Other Indirect Patient Care Areas

## INFECTION CONTROL

An Infection Control nurse gathers information regarding any type of infections in patients *and* staff members, tracks infections, and monitors infection control techniques. The Infection Control nurse teaches techniques of infection control and goes on compliance rounds, evaluating staff performance of peri care, hand-wash-

128

ing, and other Infection Control activities. S/he gathers information about infections, antibiotics, lab results relating to these infections. An Infection Control nurse may make periodic reports, tabulating the number and type of infections, and measures being taken to prevent infections. S/he may attend meetings with other department heads to discuss Infection Control issues facility-wide; for example, used dishes being left in patient rooms, laundry hampers being left open, etc.

The Infection Control Nurse must be aware of and follow state and federal guidelines regarding Infection Control.

Pros:
* day hours, no holidays or weekends
* no lifting
* use creativity in teaching about types of infections, how they are spread, and preventing infection

Cons:
* little direct patient care and contact
* conflicts between family/patient and doctor if doctor wants to treat severe infection and family does not want treatment to prolong patients life
* a lot of paperwork
* frustrating to search through chart for information

This area may be for you if:
* you enjoy paperwork
* you can assimilate and organize information from lab results, nurses notes, doctors orders, etc. to track infections
* you like to teach
* you can communicate well with doctors and other staff members to gather information and formulate a plan
* you enjoy follow-up; lab tests needed after completion of antibiotics, evaluating teaching effectiveness, continuous monitoring, etc.

This area may *not* be for you if:
* you do not enjoy paperwork
* you do not have the patience to gather information, spot a trend, formulate a plan, and follow-up
* you would rather have more direct patient contact
* you want to use technical nursing skills daily

Other information to consider:
Hospitals and Long-Term Care facilities are required to offer a yearly Infection Control/Universal Precautions inservice; the Infection Control nurse may be asked to present this inservice. An Infection Control nurse may become so familiar with teaching infection control techniques like handwashing, that she can tell, just by listening, if someone in the bathroom washes his or her hands correctly!

Skills needed:
* technical skills for collecting specimens of potentially infectious body secretions (wound cultures, sputum samples, urine)
* knowledge of, and the ability to teach, infection control techniques; hand washing, catheter care, dressing changes, etc.
* interpersonal skills to work with and teach nursing staff and staff from other departments

* * * * * * * * * * * * * * * * * * * * * *

Personal notes/comments:

## QUALITY ASSURANCE

A Quality Assurance (QA) nurse assimilates information from facility staff, residents, patients, family members, doctors, consultants, and other department personnel, to monitor and evaluate the quality and appropriateness of care provided. If there is a complaint about any aspect of care (administering medications, food quality, etc.) the QA nurse and other ancillary department personnel collect and analyze data related to the problem and brainstorm ways to resolve the problem.

If the first corrective action does not work, others will be tried. When a solution is found, periodic follow-up monitoring assures quality care continues. The QA Coordinator is in charge of directing projects and keeping track of all significant data.

Routine procedures are monitored at intervals; for example, peri care and medication administration, to assure compliance with facility policy.

130

Pros:
* day hours, no weekends or holidays
* use of creativity in solving problems
* working with a variety of people in a variety of situations
* challenging and mentally stimulating
* never boring—always working on a variety of projects
* see results of work; decrease in medication errors or increased satisfaction with admission process, for example

Cons:
* priority project(s) may change frequently
* lots of paperwork; setting up projects, collecting and analyzing data, follow-up monitoring
* may take a long time to see results

This area may be for you if:
* you like to communicate with people from all areas of the facility
* you enjoy building trust and respect between departments
* you are a good listener and can figure out what the *real* problem is
* you are very detail oriented
* you enjoy paperwork
* you can see the overall picture of how the facility needs to meet state and federal standards
* you are able to see several ways to approach and solve a problem
* you can teach, and explain projects and results

This area may *not* be for you if:
* you enjoy direct patient contact
* you don't like paperwork
* you find it difficult to gain the cooperation of personnel from other departments

Other information to consider:
Quality Assurance is a "behind the scenes" area of nursing; few people realize the work involved in maintaining standards of care, or understand "why" certain documentation is required.

Hospital personnel may expect a QA Coordinator to fix a problem *right now,* and not realize the many steps that go into analyzing and solving a problem.

Skills needed:
* basic knowledge of technical skills to identify and correct performance of procedures
* interpersonal skills for dealing with a wide variety of personalities from all departments of the facility
* leadership and management skills when organizing and completing projects

* * * * * * * * * * * * * * * * * * * *

Personal notes/comments:

## INSERVICE COORDINATOR

An Inservice Coordinator is responsible for meeting the educational requirements of all nursing department personnel, as mandated by state and federal guidelines. In small facilities, the Inservice Coordinator may also be the DON or another RN. This position may be full- or part-time.

The Inservice Coordinator is responsible for planning in-facility inservices. S/he may present the inservices personally, or ask another qualified person (who doesn't necessarily have to be a nurse) to present an inservice. The Inservice Coordinator must comply with state and federal regulations as to the number and topic of inservices presented, and s/he is responsible for keeping a record of inservices and staff attendance. The Inservice Coordinator may also teach CNA or CSM classes.

Pros:
* mainly day hours; no holidays or weekends
* can be creative in choosing topics and presenting information in fun ways
* relatively low stress job—no "life and death" situations
* usually doesn't have to wear a uniform

Cons:
- * difficult to get staff members to attend inservices; some who *do* attend make it clear they do *not* want to be at the inservice
- * tedious paperwork and record-keeping required to comply with regulations
- * may not see any direct or immediate results of your teaching
- * the Inservice Coordinator tends to have other non- related "paperwork" duties assigned
- * people asked to present an inservice may not show up at the appointed time

This area may be for you if:
- * you enjoy teaching and public speaking
- * you can make "boring" topics (infection control, universal precautions) interesting
- * direct patient care is not your priority

This area may *not* be for you if:
- * you do not like paperwork
- * you do not enjoy teaching or public speaking

Other information to consider:
An Inservice Coordinator must not take it personally if few people attend inservices, as it seems a crisis always occurs at inservice time!

Skills needed:
- * basic knowledge of technical skills so can identify and correct incorrect technique and teach new skills
- * effective teaching skills, interpersonal skills to talk with others about areas in which more education is needed,

* * * * * * * * * * * * * * * * * * * *

Personal notes/comments:

## COMPUTER (MDS Coordinator, computer programer)

As in every profession, computers are becoming more prevalent in health-care. Depending on the size of the facility, the amount of work done on a computer varies. In hospitals, it is common to use computers to track patients, and request dietary, radiology, lab, and medication orders. Some hand-held computers track vital signs and nurses notes, also. Hospitals may hire nurses to write computer programs applicable to nursing.

In a Long-Term Care facility, the MDS Coordinator gathers this information, enters it in a computer program, and sends it via modem to the state. Care Plans are formulated according to this assessment. This form, called an MDS (Minimum Data Set) gives the state information on resident cares provided, and determines the reimbursement the facility will recover from Medicaid.

Pros:
* day hours, no holidays or weekends
* no heavy lifting
* one-to-one patient contact when doing the MDS assessment
* work with co-workers from every department
* get an overall picture of a patient's/resident's condition

Cons:
* little direct patient care
* lots of time spent gathering information
* co-workers may not cooperate in providing information when needed
* co-workers may resist learning how to use computers
* problems with the computer; may take several hours to contact person who can fix it
* little use of technical nursing skills

This area may be for you if:
* you like working with computers
* you enjoy paperwork
* you like to work independently
* you enjoy assessing residents
* you are organized and detail oriented

This area may *not* be for you if:
* you do not like to work with computers

* you don't like sitting
* you do not enjoy paperwork
* you don't like working with personnel from other departments
* you would like to use technical nursing skills daily

Other information to consider:

A nurse with computer experience may be able to create and fill a new job for a facility just beginning to use computers—for example, she may enter all MDS information on the computer, or compile medication and treatment sheets.

Skills needed:
* interpersonal skills to gain the cooperation of other departments
* technical skills in working with computers

* * * * * * * * * * * * * * * * * * *

Personal notes/comments:

# Indirect Patient Care Areas
## *Out-of-Hospital*

### Director of Nursing (DON)—
### Long Term Care (LTC)

The Director of Nursing (DON) of an LTC facility is required to be an RN, and is responsible for the nurses and other nursing personnel (CNA's, CSM's), the tasks they perform, and cares they provide. S/he is ultimately responsible for all aspects of resident care. (People who reside in nursing homes are not referred to as patients, but "residents.") A DON works with all employees of the nursing department, doctors, families, and administrative personnel. S/he may be required to attend meetings and conferences.

There are many federal regulations governing LTC, and the DON is responsible for making sure regulations applicable to nursing are followed. During visits to LTC facilities, which occur at least once a year, surveyors investigate patient care areas to assure regulations are being followed. If any deficiencies in patient care are found, the DON is responsible for formulating a plan to correct the deficiency.

Pros:
* "in charge," have a lot of say about new policies, procedures, and the way the facility is run
* day hours, no scheduled weekends or holidays (unless there is a shortage of staff)
* get to know the staff members well
* opportunity to get to know residents very well and can act as a patient advocate

Cons:
* ultimately responsible for any and all nursing acts that occur in the nursing home, whether she is aware of them or not or even at the facility when they occur
* work with administration and/or a governing board who may not understand what good nursing care is and the staff, equipment, training, and supplies needed to provide good patient care

* may spend a lot of time mediating disagreements between employees (nursing and non-nursing)
* have many interruptions throughout the day, making it difficult to complete tasks and projects
* if any unit/floor/wing is short staffed on any shift, the DON may have to fill in
* can become very attached to residents, making it difficult when they die
* on call 24 hours a day, seven days a week
* you can't please everyone; someone will always be unhappy with every decision you make
* high staff turnover
* difficult to deal with budgets, especially when more staff is needed
* little opportunity to use technical nursing skills

A DON position may be for you if:
* you have a strong personality, high self-esteem, and are not bothered by negative comments about your decisions and actions
* you like the challenge of mediating disagreements between staff members
* you don't mind waiting a long time to see new policies or procedures make a difference
* you can work well with staff members from different departments, doctors, and administration
* you like to work with long-term residents and their families
* you want to try management
* you are able to be away from home if called to the facility because of an emergency
* you enjoy paperwork and are willing to follow regulations
* you are able to be flexible; work on the floor if needed, deal with emergencies

A DON position may *not* be for you if:
* you need a structured schedule without interruptions
* you are hurt by negative comments about your decisions and actions
* you like daily contact with residents
* you don't like dealing with personnel problems, which can be inconsequential
* you like to use your technical skills daily

*   you don't enjoy attending meetings

Other information:
The DON may be paid a salary or by the hour.

Generally, a DON is fairly independent. However, the scope of decisions the DON is allowed to make depends on the management style of the administrator. If you are considering a DON position, ask the administrator about his or her management style. Discuss the type of decisions you would be expected to make on your own and those on which s/he would expect to be consulted; for example, are you allowed to hire and fire nurses independently or do you need administrative approval?

Skills needed:
*   must be proficient in a wide range of assessment and technical skills; will be asked to use these skills when other nurses have questions or problems
*   interpersonal skills; working with staff members from all departments, administration, doctors, families, residents, and mediating between any or all of the above when disagreements occur; communicating with family members
*   leadership/supervisory skills; must be able to set priorities and delegate appropriately when necessary; organize projects from idea to completion and carry out the steps necessary to complete the project
*   management skills; scheduling, forming and updating care plans for each resident, infection control reports, tabulating lab results, making a budget for the nursing department, checking inventory, employee education (the DON may delegate some or all of these responsibilities, but he or she is responsible for making sure they are done correctly)

\* \* \* \* \* \* \* \* \* \* \* \* \* \* \* \* \* \* \* \*

Personal notes/comments:

# Teaching

The most obvious place in which nurses are needed to teach is colleges offering a nursing program. For nurses who don't want to make the long-term commitment to teach at a college, teaching opportunities include, Cardio Pulmonary Resuscitation (CPR), Prepared Childbirth, Certified Nursing Assistant (CNA) classes, and Care Staff Member (CSM) classes. An instructor may be required to have additional training before teaching any of the above classes.

Pros:
* pay is generally high; hours are flexible
* fairly short-term commitment; some classes may be taught for a semester (at a college), while others may meet just a few times (CPR, Prepared Childbirth)
* after preparing a lesson plan for any class, preparation time for subsequent classes is minimal
* very rewarding to help students learn a new skill, gain knowledge, and increase their self-confidence
* you can be creative in the techniques you use to teach
* work in a variety of settings when teaching nursing students—the college, various areas in the hospital and/or nursing home, community programs; also work with a variety of people—doctors, college faculty, Long-Term Care and hospital staff and community agencies
* nursing instructors teaching clinical will keep up on technical skills, and learn about new techniques, equipment, procedures, and medications

Cons:
* some students are very difficult to teach
* record keeping and grading may be tedious
* much time is required for paperwork and record keeping; preparing for classes, making and grading tests, lesson planning, student evaluations, correcting care plans, etc.

This area may be for you if:
* you are comfortable speaking in front of a group of people
* you are comfortable with your own nursing knowledge and skills
* you like to work with students

* you like to work short, fairly flexible hours
* you enjoy teaching

This area may *not* be for you if:
* you would rather perform direct patient care
* you do not like to speak in front of people or are not good at clearly explaining procedures, anatomy and physiology, the disease process, and so on
* you do not have the patience to explain things (perhaps many times!) or to watch students learn new skills
* you do not enjoy preparing for classes and the paperwork involved

Other information to consider:
Contact your local community college or university for more information about local teaching opportunities.

Skills needed:
* good base of knowledge regarding anatomy, physiology, and pathophysiology of the class subject you're teaching
* ability to demonstrate and teach technical skills
* interpersonal skills to deal with diverse personalities of students, and hospital personnel who may not be receptive to working with students
* interpersonal skills to deal with students who may not want to be in the class (taking CPR because it is required for employment), and students with various levels of education and comprehension

* * * * * * * * * * * * * * * * * * * * *

Personal notes/comments:

# Consultant

A nurse consultant can do *many* different things; consult for organizations who care for people with mental and developmental disabilities, for example. In this case, the nurse consultant may look at medication routines and teach care givers (who may not be required to be licensed and have very little training) why the medications are used and which potential side effects to closely monitor. The consultant may review medication sheets to ascertain that medications are given correctly. A nurse consultant in this case may also teach care givers how to correctly take vital signs and perform a basic assessment.

An RN may serve as a consultant to a nursing home if the nursing home is without a DON or another RN on staff. In this case, the nurse consultant could be a resource person for the staff nurses to call with questions. The consultant could also study the staffing patterns, policies, procedures, etc., and prepare a written report on any potential or actual problems and suggested solutions. Many facilities hire nurse consultants even if they have a DON, to monitor compliance with federal and state regulations and assure a good survey outcome, by their accrediting agencies.

The consultant must have knowledge of, and be willing and able to follow, state and federal laws regulating the health-care industry.

Pros:
* many opportunities to work as a consultant if you are willing to find them
* flexible hours (can usually set your own hours)
* many problems can be solved through a telephone call
* keep up-to-date on medication skills or other skills taught and used
* pay is generally high, although hours worked may vary
* varied work environments

Cons:
* may be on call 24 hours a day (although most questions can be answered over the phone)
* lots of paperwork documenting compliance with state and federal laws and regulations
* if you are working independently, you have to provide your own benefits (insurance, etc.)

This area may be for you if:
- *   you like to work independently
- *   you have good knowledge about the clients' conditions (mental retardation, epilepsy, developmental and physical disabilities) and are comfortable answering questions and teaching lay people and the clients themselves
- *   you have extensive knowledge of state and federal regulations
- *   you like to work flexible hours
- *   you don't mind paperwork and documentation

This are may *not* be for you if:
- *   you do not enjoy (or do not agree with) teaching non-licensed people how to give medications, take vital signs, etc.
- *   you enjoy working in a more structured environment (most consultants work independently)

Other information to consider:

Consultants can write much of their own job description. You may be given basic guidelines, and the freedom to implement them how you want to, as long as requirements (facility, state, federal) are met.

Consultant jobs may not be advertised. If you want to work as a consultant, develop the skills you enjoy using, such as teaching, quality assurance, monitoring medical records, etc. Offer these skills on a consultant basis. Contact the Director of Nursing at the facility at which you would like to work. For more information, talk with consultants in your area.

Skills needed:
- *   good knowledge of basic technical skills, so you can teach and monitor performance of the skills
- *   good basic knowledge of the diseases, conditions, and problems your clients are likely to have
- *   good interpersonal skills to work with various staff members
- *   confidence in yourself and your abilities, and the initiative to convince management of the need for a nurse consultant

* * * * * * * * * * * * * * * * * * * *

142

Personal notes/comments:

# State Surveyor

A State Surveyor inspects/surveys licensed health-care providers such as hospitals, Long-Term Care Units, clinics, and Home Health agencies. These facilities are inspected for compliance with Federal and State regulations regarding patient care. Surveys are completed periodically, and upon complaints by patients, staff, etc. Survey work is predominantly administrative and consultative.

Pros:
*   work mainly day hours, Monday through Friday
*   good benefits if employed full-time
*   every facility different; work is not "routine" or boring
*   opportunity to learn administrative skills
*   work with many different people
*   great chance to be a consumer/patient advocate

Cons:
*   pay usually lower than in a clinical nursing area, although if employed for a long period of time by the government, pay and benefits become substantial
*   job requires travel and possible over night (and longer) out-of-town stays
*   can be physically demanding: lots of sitting, standing, kneeling, walking necessary

This area may be for you if:
*   you have experience in clinical areas being surveyed
*   you possess excellent written communication skills
*   you have good organizational skills
*   you have exceptional interpersonal skills

This area may *not* be for you if:
*   out-of-town travel does not fit in with your lifestyle

* you do not like to use written skills; reports of up to 100 pages long may be required after surveys
* you are not comfortable confronting people (as may be necessary during a survey)

Other information about this area:

A surveyor may be required to know a second language if working in certain parts of the U.S. Personal security can be a concern when working in some areas of the U.S.

Skills needed:
* knowledge of technical skills in the clinical area surveyed
* interpersonal skills when dealing with people from every department of a facility; the ability to state problems found without making people defensive
* interpersonal skills when confronting personnel about problems found and questioning them about findings
* written communication skills when writing reports about facility findings
* organizational skills to evaluate pertinent areas of a facility
* knowledge of survey guidelines, policies and procedures

* * * * * * * * * * * * * * * * * * * *

Personal notes/comments:

# Entrepreneur—Create Your Own Perfect Job!

One of the greatest things about nursing is that career opportunities are virtually unlimited! If you haven't read about an area you think you'd enjoy, be an entrepreneur— create your own Perfect Job!

An entrepreneur must look at his or her own goals and interests, and mesh these with a "need" in nursing and/or health care.

This book was written to fill a need we heard expressed by many nurses—"I'm not happy with the job I have, but how can I find a job

144

I'll enjoy?" And so, *How to Find Your Perfect Job in Nursing* was created.

Other nurses have a special interest in a topic others know little about; working with mentally ill people who experience hallucinations, for example. One nurse made a video about the stages of hallucinations and how to work with someone having a hallucination. She also gives talks to nurses, and families of mentally ill people.

Some nurses enjoy public speaking and develop workshops related to their area of expertise. These nurses meet the need for continuing education by providing CEU's to nurses attending the workshops.

Be your own boss! The possibilities are endless!

Pros:
* you are your own boss
* opportunity to create your own Perfect Job around what you enjoy doing the most
* flexible hours—whatever hours you want to work
* high income potential

Cons:
* there may be *much* more work involved than you expect, in preparing workshops, writing a book, setting up a business, etc.
* may take a very long time to see results of your work
* may take a long time to see any financial gain
* *lots* of research necessary to write, give talks, provide CEU's, start a business
* start-up money may be necessary

Entrepreneurship may be for you if:
* you are highly motivated, willing to do the work involved to identify a need and fill it

Entrepreneurship may *not* be for you if:
* you need the security of a job in which you know what is expected of you, and what you will be doing each day

Other information about being an entrepreneur:
An entrepreneur must be *very* motivated, creative, and a self-starter. When you are in business for yourself, there is no one to tell you when to go to work, what to do next, etc. *You* have to be the

145

one to take the initiative to create your own success. The amount of time and work involved in finding your "niche" is tremendous! A supportive family can make the process less stressful.

Skills needed:
* thorough knowledge of the area you are writing about, speaking about, etc.
* organization, motivation, the ability to be your own cheer-leader

* * * * * * * * * * * * * * * * * * * * *

Personal notes/comments:

# Federal Employment Nursing Opportunities

There are numerous civilian and active duty nursing positions available within the Federal Government. The Civil Service Administration staffs civilian nurses in the military base hospital facilities and the Veterans Administration needs civilian nurses to staff the numerous Veteran Administration Hospitals and Long-Term Care facilities throughout the United States. In addition to these nursing positions, there are also positions and careers awaiting nurses in the U.S. Navy, U.S. Air Force, and U.S. Army, with some select nursing positions available in the Reserves of these military branches. While it is impossible to describe every position available, as they are so diverse, there are many generalized statements and comparisons which may be helpful.

*Civilian:* Civil Service jobs require meeting the minimum requirement for the job description of the *open* position you are currently seeking (you cannot apply for any job that is not open). You must first pass a test which is scored by points and then adjusted to reflect your experience, skill level, and years of service to the Federal Government. Higher test-scoring applicants can get passed over by lower test-scoring applicants in this system. Depending on your

146

total points, you are ranked and are either eligible or ineligible for selection. It is not uncommon to be eligible and passed over for selection the first time you apply! Perseverance pays off! Civil Service openings do not necessarily require a BSN.

Beginning salaries are usually not as competitive as jobs in other health care facilities, but continued employment and job reviews enable the competent nurse to receive routine "step" pay raises as well as excellent federal employee benefit packages. These nurses are usually very satisfied with their employment.

As in the private sector, the military is now scaling down, which also affects the Civil Service employment needs. The Civil Service nurse finds it in his or her best interest, as do *all* nurses today, to cross-train to make themselves more marketable in any employment realm.

For any information regarding current federal employment and career opportunities, call the Career America Connection at (912) 757-3000. You will receive information regarding special programs for students, Veterans, the disabled, the Presidential Management Intern Program, and Salaries and Benefits. All requested information is mailed within 24 hours. If you have a computer, scan online by calling the Federal Job Opportunity Board at (912) 757-3100. For specific job openings within the VA, call (800) 942-0002, The Office of Health Care Recruitment and Development. Your Perfect Job may be just a phone call away!

*Active Duty:* The United States Air Force (USAF), United States Army, and United States Navy are all currently actively recruiting nurses. These openings are more competitive than in previous years and all do require a minimum educational level of a BSN, as well as a three to four year commitment to active duty. All branches commission their BSN's as officers, and all require attendance to a basic indoctrination specific to their respective branches, to learn history, custom and traditions, rank recognition, military etiquette, personnel management, etc. The nurses do *not* attend "Basic Training" with its' stringent physical regime, although physical fitness remains a top priority.

The current fiscal year's funding has allowed Air Force and Navy more recruitment slots, with Army able to only enlist the following specific areas of nursing: Nurse Anesthetists, Family Nurse Practitioners, and *experienced* Critical Care RN's. This will remain the same for Army through September of 1997.

All three branches offer educational assistance to students in a BSN level and higher prior to active duty; however, due to the Army's current fiscal funding and specifications of active enlistments, this assistance cannot be extended to nurses enlisting requiring assistance with a BSN. It would, however, be able to assist with education for a Master's level and higher, for those nurses enlisting this year, who meet the specialties criteria above. Therefore, prior to Oct. 1997, new and existing BSN graduates and students needing employment or educational assistance for 1997 and 1998 should contact the local Navy or Air Force Recruiter for more specific details.

There seems to be a gross misconception regarding relocation and assignment of military nurses in peace-time. All three branches report that it is customarily a volunteer assignment on overseas peace-keeping missions (unless not enough volunteer in any given specialty).

As with Civil Service, beginning salaries alone are not competitive with general clinical salaries, but with rank and continued years of service, as well as the benefit packages available, they do exceed the private sector down the road.

Pros:
* great educational opportunity with educational assistance provided by the service
* opportunity to travel
* work in a variety of settings
* meet professionals from throughout the United States— and world!
* great benefits and retirement benefits
* promotion chances good

Cons:
* may require deployment on short notice, requiring separation from family
* may have conflict with a superior and trouble gaining reassignment
* positions on active duty are *competitive*— employees don't always get the position they want

This area may be for you if:
* you like change
* you enjoy travelling
* you have a sense of adventure!

This area may *not* be for you if:
* you find it difficult to follow orders
* you do not like to travel

* * *

*"The Navy has fantastic opportunities for travel all over the world!"*
                    Anne Burke, RN, former U.S. Navy Nurse
                    U.S. Navy 1-800-USA-NAVY


*"What I like about nursing in the Army is that I'm not only taking care of patients, but people who are serving their country. I find that particularly rewarding."*
                    Capt. Neva Westhoff, (RN)
                    U.S. Army 1-800-USA-ARMY


*"There are incredible opportunities for nurses in the Air Force with all the diverse roles to pursue."*
                    Major Carol Amadeo, RN
                    U.S. Air Force (402) 291-7424

# Interest List:

**AREAS IN WHICH I HAVE *SOME* INTEREST;**
**AREAS IN WHICH I HAVE A *STRONG* INTEREST**

As you read through the job descriptions in this section, jot down areas in which you have some interest, and areas in which you have a strong interest in working. Also record the page number on which the information begins—then you'll be able to find pertinent information when preparing for an interview.

| Areas in which I have *some* interest | Page | Areas in which I have a *strong* interest | Page |
|---|---|---|---|
| | | | |

# Skills Utilization Checklist

After you determine the skills you are interested in using in your Perfect Job, you may use this checklist as a quick reference to see in which jobs your strengths will be utilized.

K =level of Knowledge needed for the specific skills area
     * = basic level of knowledge needed
    ** = intermediate level of knowledge needed
  *** = advanced level of knowledge needed

U =amount of time spent actually Using the specific skills area
     * = rarely or never used
    ** = skills used daily
  *** = skills used several times daily

| CLINICAL AREA | TECHNICAL SKILLS | INTER-PERSONAL SKILLS | LEADER-SHIP SKILLS | MANAGE-MENT SKILLS |
|---|---|---|---|---|
| **Direct Patient Care In-Hospital** | | | | |
| Med/Surg— General | K ** <br> U *** | K ** <br> U ** | K * <br> U * | K * <br> U * |
| Med/Surg— Specialty | K *** <br> U *** | K ** <br> U ** | K * <br> U * | K * <br> U * |
| Out-Patient Services | K *** <br> U *** | K ** <br> U *** | K * <br> U * | K * <br> U * |
| Emergency Room | K *** <br> U *** | K *** <br> U *** | K * <br> U * | K * <br> U * |
| Operating Room | K *** <br> U *** | K * <br> U * | K * <br> U * | K * <br> U * |
| Recovery/ PACU | K *** <br> U *** | K ** <br> U ** | K * <br> U * | K * <br> U * |

151

| | | | | |
|---|---|---|---|---|
| CC/ICU/PICU | K *** | K *** | K * | K * |
| | U *** | U *** | U * | U * |
| Rehab-ilitation | K ** | K *** | K * | K * |
| | U ** | U *** | U * | U * |
| Psychiatric | K ** | K *** | K * | K * |
| | U * | U *** | U * | U * |
| Labor and Delivery | K *** | K *** | K * | K * |
| | U *** | U *** | U * | U * |
| Post-partum | K ** | K *** | K * | K * |
| | U ** | U *** | U * | U * |
| Newborn Nursery | K *** | K ** | K * | K * |
| | U ** | U ** | U * | U * |
| Pediatrics | K *** | K *** | K * | K * |
| | U *** | U *** | U * | U * |
| Transplant | K *** | K *** | K * | K * |
| | U *** | U *** | U * | U * |
| Hemodialysis Acute | K *** | K *** | K * | K * |
| | U *** | U *** | U * | U * |
| Cardiac Rehab | K *** | K ** | K * | K * |
| | U * | U ** | U * | U * |

## Direct Patient Care—
## Out-of Hospital

| | | | | |
|---|---|---|---|---|
| Long-term Care | K *** | K *** | K * | K * |
| | U ** | U *** | U * | U * |
| Home Health | K *** | K *** | K * | K * |
| | U ** | U *** | U * | U * |

| | | | | |
|---|---|---|---|---|
| Hospice | K *** <br> U ** | K *** <br> U *** | K * <br> U * | K * <br> U * |
| Clinic/ Dr's. Office | K *** <br> U * | K *** <br> U ** | K * <br> U * | K * <br> U * |
| Occupational/ Industrial | K ** <br> U * | K ** <br> U ** | K * <br> U * | K * <br> U * |
| Hemodialysis Chronic | K *** <br> U ** | K ** <br> U ** | K * <br> U * | K * <br> U * |
| Traveling | K *** <br> U *** | K *** <br> U *** | K * <br> U * | K * <br> U * |
| Prison | K *** <br> U *** | K *** <br> U *** | K * <br> U * | K * <br> U * |
| Private Duty | K *** <br> U ** | K *** <br> U *** | K * <br> U * | K * <br> U * |
| School | K *** <br> U ** | K *** <br> U *** | K * <br> U * | K * <br> U * |
| Camp | K *** <br> U * | K *** <br> U *** | K * <br> U * | K * <br> U * |
| Flight | K *** <br> U *** | K ** <br> U ** | K * <br> U * | K * <br> U * |
| Insurance Exams | K * <br> U * | K *** <br> U *** | K * <br> U * | K * <br> U * |
| Armed Forces | K *** <br> U *** | K *** <br> U *** | K *** <br> U *** | K ** <br> U ** |
| Parish | K * <br> U * | K *** <br> U *** | K ** <br> U ** | K * <br> U * |
| Bloodmobile | K *** <br> U *** | K ** <br> U ** | K * <br> U * | K * <br> U * |

## Indirect Patient Care—
## In-hospital

| | | | | |
|---|---|---|---|---|
| Team Leader | K ***<br>U ** | K ***<br>U *** | K ***<br>U *** | K *<br>U * |
| Charge Nurse | K ***<br>U ** | K ***<br>U *** | K ***<br>U *** | K *<br>U * |
| Head Nurse | K ***<br>U ** | K ***<br>U *** | K ***<br>U *** | K **<br>U * |
| DON-Hospital | K ***<br>U * | K ***<br>U *** | K ***<br>U *** | K ***<br>U *** |
| ADON | K ***<br>U * | K ***<br>U *** | K ***<br>U *** | K ***<br>U *** |
| House Supervisor | K ***<br>U * | K ***<br>U *** | K ***<br>U *** | K ***<br>U *** |
| Infection Control | K **<br>U * | K ***<br>U *** | K **<br>U ** | K *<br>U * |
| Quality Assurance | K **<br>U * | K ***<br>U *** | K **<br>U ** | K *<br>U * |
| Inservice Coordinator | K ***<br>U * | K ***<br>U *** | K *<br>U * | K *<br>U * |
| Computer | K ***<br>U * | K **<br>U ** | K *<br>U * | K *<br>U * |

## Indirect Patient Care—
## Out of Hospital

| | | | | |
|---|---|---|---|---|
| D.O.N.—Long-Term Care | K ***<br>U * | K ***<br>U *** | K ***<br>U *** | K ***<br>U *** |

| | | | | |
|---|---|---|---|---|
| Teaching | K *** | K *** | K ** | K * |
| | U * | U *** | U ** | U * |
| Consultant | K *** | K *** | K * | K * |
| | U ** | U *** | U * | U * |
| State Surveyors | K *** | K *** | K * | K *** |
| | U * | U *** | U * | U ** |
| Entrepreneur | K *** | K *** | K *** | K *** |
| | U * | U *** | U * | U ** |
| Federal Employment | K *** | K *** | K ** | K ** |
| | U *** | U *** | U ** | U ** |

-------------------------------------------------------------------------

*"Talk to someone who works in that area. Work on-call for awhile before taking a full-time job."* Linda Edelman, R.N.

# SECTION THREE

# Landing Your Perfect Job

*"In all jobs I believe a formal mentor is important. Someone who helps you grow, who offers constructive criticism."* Jean Beyer, R.N.

# How to Use This Section

Congratulations! You've defined your Perfect Job, researched many areas of nursing—now we'll show you how to go out and win your Perfect Job!

This section takes you through the actual job-hunting process, from writing your resume to the first days on your new job. We've included several worksheets which you will find extremely valuable; make copies of them if you need to. Read this section completely before you begin your job search, so you can quickly locate the information you need at any given point of the job-hunting process.

# Tracking Down Your Perfect Job

At first glance, it may seem like your Perfect Job is not available in your area—or is it? You have checked the want ads, listed with your local Job Service, and even called the personnel manager of facilities of interest to you, but to no avail. There are still areas you should explore before just scrapping your vision of your Perfect Job (and settling for what is apparently readily available), or even starting to consider relocation—unless, of course, relocation is an option!

This is where having tenacity and good interpersonal skills becomes invaluable. Many "good" and desirable jobs are not even advertised. During the research for this book, we contacted the local Job Service and used their computer to conduct a search of nursing jobs available nationwide. According to this computer, there were only 252 nursing jobs available—nationwide—in general, specialty, and management areas! Anyone with even the vaguest idea of the status of nursing vacancies knows that this is not an accurate reflection of jobs unfilled!

This is when and where *you* take control of your destiny in the quest for your Perfect Job! A good way to continue your search is to network with the nurses you know, especially those working in facilities in which you would enjoy working. Talk with your doctor, his or her nurses, and any other nurses you know. Tell them you are looking for a job and ask them if they know of any openings. Keep in contact with your Job Service interviewer; s/he may not have been given a complete listing of jobs available in the area, but may be able to provide valuable information on how to make opportunities available to you.

For example, a close friend of ours had over 20 years of experience in various areas of critical care. After taking a break from nursing while her children were babies, she was eager to work again. She polished her resume to perfection, and had an outstanding work history and references. By following the guidance in this book, she defined her Perfect Job. As she had small children at home, a Monday through Friday day-shift job was a priority. She did not want to commute more than 40 miles each way. She was open to what clinical area she wanted to work in and whether she worked full-or part-time.

She then targeted her resume (as will be discussed), registered with the job service, and hand delivered her resume to all facilities offering Monday through Friday day hours, within a 40 mile radius of her home. She scoured the want ads daily, and in three months found only one ad fitting her Perfect Job description. At one time the applicant thought she had located the perfect job—35 miles from home, day hours with weekends and holidays off—but the facility offered only twelve-hour shifts. With the commute, our friend would be gone 14 hours and that simply did not fit her Perfect Job description. Reluctantly, she turned down the job. She knew that even as badly as she wanted it, if she took it, eventually both she *and* her employer would be unhappy.

When she called to turn down the job, she stated her reason why and asked if eight-hour shifts were available in any areas in the facility. From the networking she had done, the applicant had discovered that eight-hour shifts were usually available on certain outpatient units. She mentioned this to the Personnel Director, stressing her long history of excellent IV and assessment skills. The manager sent her an application, which the employee filled out and returned the next day, along with another copy of her resume.

About this time, the applicant was getting frustrated with all of her hard work—and still no Perfect Job! The Job Service then made another valuable suggestion; call directly to the department head of the area in which you are seeking a job. By calling the switchboard at the hospital and asking for the Charge Nurse on the Hemodialysis Unit, our friend was transferred to the right person! She introduced herself, briefly stated her credentials and experience, and asked if any positions were available. Pay dirt at last! The applicant was informed of the need for a part-time nurse on the day shift! The Charge Nurse stated she would locate the applicant's resume and set up an interview for the next week! With her professional (and tenacious) attitude, the applicant was very well received. Even though she had no Hemodialysis experience, her experience in critical care more than qualified her for the job.

So you see, it pays to be persistent. Very few jobs are actually advertised in the want ads; most are filled through word of mouth and determination of someone who really wants to find his or her Perfect Job. With a professional attitude and perseverance, you too will find your Perfect Job—if not directly, through a "friend who knows a friend . . ." This applicant found success because she narrowed down her Target Area and knew what her Perfect Job was—and was willing to work for it.

# Writing the Perfect Resume

For every good nursing position open, you can be sure that numerous qualified people will apply. How, then, do you make *your* resume stand out from the others? First of all, you must decide how badly you want a particular job. You must want the job badly enough to take the time to write a resume with a specific job in mind—not just a "generic" resume that could be used when applying for any job from Labor and Delivery to Hospice to Critical Care. The process of individually preparing a resume for a specific job is, of course, time consuming (and can be expensive), especially when you are writing several carefully worded resumes for jobs within your Target Area(s). However, you can simplify the process and still provide an impressive resume unique to the position for which you have applied.

By now you should know what specific jobs are available, for which you wish to apply. You have determined, from the Skills Utilization Checklist on page 151 exactly what skills are needed for these specific jobs. Write down each job for which you are applying, and the skills utilized in each job. Draft a resume emphasizing your qualifications unique to these skills. State your "added values," that is, extra training or skill you have in these areas. For example, in an area which emphasizes teaching skills, note your experience presenting an inservice or preparing patient education materials. For a position in a clinical area which requires excellent interpersonal skills, point out workshops you have attended or research you've done in this area. For a position requiring leadership skills, document any committees you've served on (even if not in a healthcare setting). Show qualifications that are unique to *you* and will exceed the level of experience of the average applicant.

See, you have just created a winning resume, easily modified to apply to more than one specific position! Thanks to the wonders of modern technology, it is now possible to reach a vast audience of potential employers by posting your resume on the Internet. This free service for healthcare recruitment is on the MedSearch America Internet site at:

http://www.medsearch.com.

For more information about writing resumes, we suggest *The Damn Good Resume Guide* by Yana Parker and *Power Resumes* by Ron Tepper. These, and other guides, can be found in your bookstore or local library.

Remember—the most important thing you can do when preparing your resume is to demonstrate mastery of the required skills and define your "added values." This, more often than not, will win you the interview that will lead to your Perfect Job in Nursing!

# Making the Interview Work for You

As expected, your resume generated several appointments for interviews. Your mind is probably racing ahead to planning your wardrobe and getting a manicure to assure that "good first impression." There are many factors that influence the successfulness of the interview—from the standpoint of the interviewer as well as that of the interviewee—that is, you.

The very first impression you give may be your completed job application, which, at some point during the job-hunting process, you will be required to complete. If possible, complete the application *before* the interview, so you can take your time and make sure it is filled out neatly, accurately, and completely.

The completed job application gives a wealth of information about the applicant. Supervisors, administrators, and others in a hiring position, form their first opinion about applicants from the completed application. Make sure the job application is filled out *completely*—leave *no* blank spaces. Every application has a space for the applicant's signature; some facilities purposely use forms on which this space is difficult to find. At a glance, they can see if the applicant has paid attention to detail and signed the application; if it is not signed, the applicant is immediately disqualified. Make sure your application makes a great first impression—it can be your key to landing that all-important interview!

We have divided the interview process into three parts. "Pre-Interview" gives suggestions on preparing for the interview, "Peri-Interview" discusses hints for the interview itself, and "Post-Interview" dissects the interview and gives you information on rating the interview and perhaps improving the process next time. Use the "Employment Follow-up Tracking Sheet" on page 175 to keep track of what point you are at in the interview and follow-up process of each job for which you have applied.

*Pre-Interview*

Your first contact with the interviewer (who may be your potential boss!) may be over the telephone, when you call to inquire about available jobs, or a specific job advertised. During this initial contact, observe basic phone etiquette; minimize interruptions (bribe the kids to be quiet, if necessary!), speak clearly, and at the beginning of the conversation, introduce yourself and briefly state the nature of your call.

Some employers conduct "mini-interviews" over the phone as an initial screening process, so be prepared to answer questions about your education, experience, and position desired.

Before the call, make a list of questions *you* need answered—specifics of job(s) available, the area, shift(s), etc. If an interview is scheduled, write down the date, time, and location, along with directions for getting there. Write down the specifics in several places—never rely on your memory for information this important!

Even if you sense, through the phone call, that jobs available at that facility are not for you, you may choose to go to the interview anyway. The job may turn out to be your Perfect Job, and even if not, you will have knowledge of the facility, should another position become available in the future. You will also have a chance to practice and perfect your interview skills. However, if after the interview, you have no intention of even considering the job, it is not fair to give the interviewer the impression that you *would* consider an offer. Thank the interviewer for his or her time and state that you feel the job just would not work for you. Send a thank-you note, and if appropriate, state that you would consider a position in the future.

While it is always wise to look your best for an interview (good hygiene and impeccably clean, professional attire are always your best bets), it is also short-sighted to believe that these factors alone influence the interviewer's first impression. A pleasant facial expression, direct eye contact, a firm handshake, and good interpersonal skills are also being considered, as are your other less obvious body language signals. To establish rapport with your interviewer, follow his or her lead; sit when asked to, make small talk, and if the interviewer makes a joke which you find humorous, smile and laugh.

However good your resume, first impression, and interpersonal skills may be, there is still more to do to win your desired job offer. Seasoned interviewers are looking for certain criteria in potential employees. And while we are all aware of the above mentioned generic criteria, the interviewers also have specific criteria for each position for which they are interviewing.

To determine the interviewer's specific criteria for the "perfect person," politely ask the interviewer if s/he will answer a few questions, before the interview actually begins, to enable you to address these areas of mutual interest throughout the interview. Ask questions about the job available, and request a job description up front. By establishing this specific criteria at the beginning of the interview, you are able to "sell" yourself to these particular aspects of the job. By stating your "added value", that is, focusing on your unique strengths that will make you a valuable employee in this position, you will leave a very positive impression on the interviewer.

There are several excellent books you can refer to as resources for the interview process; *The Five-Minute Interview* by Richard H. Beatty; *Getting to the Right Job* by Steve Cohen and Paulo deOlivera; and *Ready, Aim, You're Hired!* by Paul Hellman. If you feel ill-prepared, or nervous about the interview process, utilize the expert advice available. Your comfort level with the interview process is *vital* to a positive outcome. We have found that the most successful way to overcome pre-interview jitters is by being well-practiced and well- prepared. We suggest that you write out the questions you deem most significant (suggestions listed on the next page) and then practice saying them out loud to familiarize yourself with your chosen wording. Again, you want to be comfortable with the questions you wish to ask, as well as replies to the questions you expect to be asked.

The interview is not only an opportunity for the interviewer to evaluate *you*, but also gives you a chance to check out the facility which may be your future work home.

Below is a list of sample questions which we feel would be of great benefit to ask during an interview for *any* nursing job. Any of these questions should help you better understand the job expectations.

## Question to Ask During the Interview

1. Why is this job open?

2. What are the primary responsibilities of this job? May I see a job description? (this gives you a clear picture of what your responsibilities and duties would be)

3. What is the facility mission statement?

4. What was the outcome of the last facility survey? May I see a copy of the last survey and any deficiencies cited? Has a plan of correction been completed and implemented?
   (Surveys are done periodically by various regulatory and accrediting agencies to assure patient care is adequately provided; the answer to these questions will give you an idea of any problems within the facility. Nurses in management positions are expected to resolve these problems.)

5. What is the administration's philosophy toward Nursing Services?

6.  What is the administrator's (or your supervisor's) management style?
    (Are nurses allowed to make independent decisions, or are they required to check with management before making changes?)

7.  What is your orientation for new nurses? (Do you feel certain that you could function confidently after the orientation outlined?)

List other questions *you* want to ask in the space below.

Again, these are just examples to nudge your thinking. These questions may, or may not, pertain to your specific job interview. Your goal is to formulate questions that are applicable to your particular Perfect Job, and will supply you with the best insight to the employer's needs and philosophies. By diligently working on these questions prior to your interview, you will have optimized your advantage to sell your education, qualifications, skills, and added values. Remember, the information obtained is only as good as the questions you ask! Therefore, the initial questions you prepare are equivalent to the end result of your interview.

You will be expected to provide pertinent information regarding your nursing education, experiences, and any previous employment. By reviewing your dates of employment, and by reflecting on any lapses of employment, and the circumstances pertaining to such, or any job changes, you should be able to respond to these questions in a candid, yet informative way. Do keep in mind, it is never wise to volunteer any negative past job experience(s). But it is also best to be prepared to speak briefly regarding any negative aspects of your employment history, should the need arise. If there are less desirable aspects of your employment history, or qualifications, be prepared to have a response that will show the interviewer how the problem has been corrected, or how other experiences or skills can help offset any possible deficit they may note regarding your potential employment. Often a willing and eager attitude to learn will convince a potential employer that *you* are the person worth training!

The questions below are some of the most commonly asked at interviews. Please utilize the space below each question to formulate your personal responses.

* Why did you choose a career in nursing?

* Why did you apply at this facility?

* How did you hear about this job?

* Why are you applying for this job?

* What are your qualifications for this job?

* What are your strengths?

* How will you utilize these strengths in this job?

* What are your weaknesses or limitations?

* How will you improve on your weaknesses or compensate for your limitations?

* Where do you see yourself in 1, 2, and 5 years?

* Will you have difficulty working the scheduled hours as described?

* If I were to call your references, what do you think they would tell me?

* What are your salary expectations and requirements?

* Will your health preclude you from performing the job you are applying for, based upon the job description?

* How has your past employment attendance been?

* What specialized skills can you perform? Do you have documentation of these skills?

* And, the most dreaded, "Tell me about yourself." (They *don't* need to know about your pitiful love-life or any emotional scars left from childhood; they are interested in hearing about accomplishments, motivation, professional affiliations and accomplishments, community involvements, etc.—this is your time to brag!)

Certainly, other questions will be asked, but by reviewing these basic questions you should be able to proficiently respond to any other questions that may come your way. You are now ready to impress your interviewer with your dazzling, insightful answers!

So, review the checklists below, then relax with the knowledge that you're well prepared!

# Pre-Interview Checklist

The following checklists will help you make the best first impression possible.

### Pre-interview checklist:

YES    NO

1. Do you have pre-interview questions prepared to ask the interviewer? Do you have follow-up questions and answers prepared?

2. Are you comfortable with how you will phrase the above questions and answers?

3. Have you reviewed your past job history and can you recall dates and situations without difficulty?

4. Have you reviewed your "Interest Assessment" (page 57), "Things to Observe During the Tour," (below), and "Unit Dynamics" (page 183)?

5. Have you identified your added values and strengths, and considered ways to apply them to the job?

6. Have you organized your personal accessories, portfolio, etc.? (so no coupons fall out of your purse at an inopportune time or you are unable to locate your pen or nursing license)

7.  Have you selected a clean, professional outfit and accessories for the interview?

8.  Have you maximized your personal appearance by having good personal hygiene, with clean and neatly styled hair, fresh manicure, polished shoes, etc.?

9.  Do you know how to get to the interview location and have you allowed adequate driving time?

10. Do you know the name of the person conducting the interview?

11. Have you answered "yes" to all of the above questions?

If your answer to number 11 is "no", you are not ready for the interview and need more preparation. If your answer to number 11 is "yes" proceed to gather the items necessary to make a positive impression, as listed below.

Suggested items to take with you:

*   several copies of your resume, in case your interviewer does not have one
*   your nursing license or other paperwork to verify your credentials
*   your list of pre-interview questions, and other questions you want to ask
*   a file folder, portfolio, or briefcase to hold all paperwork
*   a pen that works (black ink is most professional)
*   an extra pair of pantyhose, safety pins, etc.
*   explicit directions to the place of the interview
*   breath mints or gum (remove before the interview begins)
*   tissues in pocket

The most important thing to do during the interview itself is to relax and be yourself! If you have a habit of fidgeting, make an effort to be aware of this and minimize it as much as possible during the interview.

Do let your true personality show through. Don't be afraid to smile, nod in agreement, or even laugh if it is appropriate to the situation. If the interviewer asks you a difficult question, take a deep breath and collect your thoughts before you answer.

Remember to ask the questions *you* have about the job or facility. Do this at appropriate times during the interview, and don't be afraid to jot down pertinent answers, so you can refer to the information later.

If you will need time off during the next three months or so (for a wedding, or trip that has already been planned), inform your potential employer of that. Before you consider a job offer, you will have to be sure that you can get the time off. This may seem presumptuous, but you don't want to place yourself in the position of having to negotiate time off when you've just been hired! After all, vacation days are usually not available to use for several months.

At some point during or after your interview, you will probably tour the facility-or at least the floor or area in which you will work, if you are offered the job. If the interviewer does not offer to take you on a tour, by all means, request one! You certainly want to evaluate the setting and atmosphere of your potential Perfect Job!

The tour gives you a wonderful opportunity to evaluate the facility as a whole, the area/floor in which you may be working, and the people you could be working with. Jot down your impressions after the interview and consider them in your decision whether or not to accept a job offer.

*Things to Observe During the Tour*

The facility itself: Is it clean? Well kept? Is the paint chipped? Wallpaper scuffed? Tiles loose? Is there a fresh smell, or a "hospital" or "Long-term Care" odor?

The floor on which you may be working:
Are there a lot of call bells/call lights on? Do medication/report/charting areas and the nursing station appear organized, or cluttered and disorganized? Is the area/floor, as a whole, clean and neat? Are there cartoons and jokes as well as memos, rules, and regulations posted on bulletin boards? Try to sense the atmosphere and mood; is it tense? relaxed? friendly?

People throughout the facility and in the specific area in which you might be working:
Do people smile and say "hello" whether or not they are introduced to you? Do the nurses appear calm (A nurse can be calm *and* busy) or harassed? Do co-workers speak kindly and politely to each other? To patients? On the telephone?

Remember—anyone can have a bad day, which would give a negative impression. However, if almost everyone seems harried or unfriendly, the area may have many nurses with personality conflicts or unresolved issues. A comfortable work atmosphere is synonymous with your job compatibility.

Towards the end of the interview, review the list of questions you have prepared for the interviewer and be sure they have all been answered. After the interview, thank the interviewer for taking the time to talk with you. If an offer has not been extended, ask the interviewer when you can expect to hear from them regarding the job.

*Post-interview*

As soon as you return to your car, jot down your impressions of the interview and facility. Also record any responses to the questions you asked, and other pertinent information. The day of the interview, or the day after at the latest, write a brief note of appreciation to each interviewer who took the time to meet with you.

Now take time to reflect on your interview performance. Overall, were you satisfied? Were there areas you feel needed more polish? Did the interviewer ask questions that you were not prepared to answer? Make a note for future reference and clip it to your personal copy of your resume, and prepare better in those areas prior to any future interviews.

Always complete the interview process. For instance, if you interviewed for three jobs, but had only two employment offers, place a call or write a letter to the interviewer who did not extend a job offer. Ask for a brief critique of your qualifications, resume, and interview performance. Let the person know you are genuinely interested in his or her opinion and welcome input on which areas to improve for future interviews. Again, take notes to clip to your personal copy of your resume. Always thank the interviewer for any input, regardless of the outcome. There may come a time you will interview with this person again, and they will recall how you valued their opinion. There is a universal truth to the philosophy that you should never burn a bridge . . .

Lastly, relax, clear your mind, objectively compile all the information you have gathered (don't forget your "gut feelings"), and fill in the "Job Offer Comparison Worksheet" on page 176 to assist you in your final decision.

# My Perfect Job Worksheet

From the quizzes, worksheets, and information presented in Section One, indicate your Perfect Job specifics in the appropriate area below.

* * *

Summarize personal needs and goals as related to your Perfect Job: (from pages 6-7)


Summarize family needs and goals as related to your Perfect Job: (from pages 8-9)


Summarize career needs and goals as related to your Perfect Job: (from pages 10-11)

* * *

Priority benefits (from pages 15-16)
    1.        4.
    2.        5.
    3.

* * *

(from page 22)

| Willing to commute | | Willing to commute if: |
|---|---|---|
| 1-10 miles | less than 10 minutes | (conditions) |
| 11-25 miles | 10-30 minutes | |
| 26-40 miles | 31-60 minutes | |
| 40+ miles | 61+ minutes | |

Not willing to commute

\* \* \*

(from page 26)         Full-time         Part-time ____hours per week

\* \* \*

(from page 34)         Day shift         Evening shift   Night shift

   Twelve-hour days  Twelve-hour nights      Short shifts

\* \* \*

(from page 36)         Small facility   Large facility   No preference

\* \* \*

(from page 38)         Direct patient care      Indirect patient care
                              No preference

\* \* \*

(from page 42)         General nursing          Specialty area

\* \* \*

(from page 47)         Primary nursing          Team nursing

\* \* \*

(from page 56)         Technical skills         Interpersonal skills
      Leadership skills          Management skills

\* \* \*

My top priorities are:         I am willing to compromise on:

# Employment Follow-Up Tracking Sheet

| FACILITY NAME, ADDRESS, PHONE | DATE RESUME SENT AND TO WHOM | DATE OF INITIAL PHONE CONTACT AND WITH WHOM | FOLLOW-UP PERSON AND DATE | FOLLOW-UP CONTACTS | COMMENTS |
|---|---|---|---|---|---|
| | | | | | |

# Job Offer Comparison Worksheet

*What is your Perfect Job? "One that is stimulating to your mind, yet does not drain your energy, so you can also have a personal life . . . "* Kathy Engel, R.N.

*"Trust your gut feelings."* Anita Kaspar, L.P.N.

\* \* \*

Fill in information about each job you are offered; it will be easy to see any information you need to collect.

| | JOB #1 | JOB #2 | JOB #3 | JOB #4 |
|---|---|---|---|---|
| **Facility name** | | | | |
| **Nursing area** | | | | |
| **Shift offered** | | | | |
| **Hours per week** | | | | |
| **Pay per hour** | | | | |
| COMPARISON FACTORS | | | | |
| How job fits needs & goals: personal | | | | |
| family | | | | |
| career | | | | |
| Priority benefits: | | | | |
| 1. | | | | |
| 2. | | | | |
| 3. | | | | |
| 4. | | | | |
| 5. | | | | |

Offered by
   facility?

Commute

Strengths
utilized in
this job

Are they the
strengths you
want to use?

Impression of:
   facility
   work area
   personnel in
   work area
   all personnel

Gut instinct,
other info

# Before You Accept *Any* Job Offer . . .

*"Talk to nurses and ask for honest feelings—visit different areas at different times of shifts."* Katherine Smith, R.N.

You did it! You defined your Perfect Job, wrote a wonderful resume, impressed everyone during your interview, and received a job offer! Congratulations!

But wait—before you accept the job offer, you still have several things to do to make certain *this* job is Your Perfect Job in Nursing.

During the job offer call, confirm the specifics of the job you are being offered (shift, area, pay, etc.) and ask any questions you may have—about benefits, orientation, and so on. Ask for several days to consider the offer, and set up a date and time to call and give your answer.

During this time interval, follow up on all potential Perfect Job opportunities. (you should be tracking potential Perfect Jobs on your Employment Follow-up Tracking Sheet). Have all contacts returned necessary calls? Have you contacted all facilities? It's OK to tell other prospects that you have received an offer and wanted to see if they had made a decision regarding your employment.

To assess if the job you've been offered *is* in fact, your Perfect Job, you need some quiet time. Imagine yourself actually going to the job you have been offered. Picture yourself walking through the door, performing nursing activities, and interacting with the people you've met. What is your gut feeling? Is the job right for you? If you are considering several job offers, visualize them as above. Does any one or several feel wrong for you? Your Job Comparison Worksheet will further help you determine which will be the Perfect Job. If you are *still* debating between several jobs, make a list of pros and cons of each job. Your Perfect Job should be clear.

If it is *still* not clear, pretend for a few minutes that you have made the decision to accept one of the jobs. How do you feel? Doubtful? Relieved?

After completing these exercises, you should know, beyond any shadow of a doubt, which job is your Perfect Job. If not, you need to collect more pertinent information before you make your decision. Review the information you have, and fill in any gaps, either from your own knowledge or after calling the facility.

Notify the facility (or facilities) of your decision as soon as you've made it. Don't be afraid of saying you're turning down a job offer; if you made a good impression during your contacts with the facility, you will be remembered in a positive way, should you apply for another position in the future. If your ex-potential employer is overtly upset at your decision to turn down the job, you've learned a valuable lesson—that you made the right decision! When you call to accept your Perfect Job, be sure to findout to whom, and when and where you should report for orientation, and what you should wear.

Now—relax, and celebrate! Spread the word! Brag a little (or a lot)! You've just found Your Perfect Job in Nursing!

# Making The First Days On Your New, Perfect Job, Easier

*"Get as much experience as you can and be open to new opportunities."* Anne Burke, R.N.

Even experienced nurses have anxiety those first few days on a new job. Although you may be comfortable with basic procedures, policies for performing those procedures, such as ordering X-rays, or transcribing doctors orders, are different at each facility. And different floors within the same hospital may have unique routines and store necessary supplies in unexpected places.

For students and new grads, your first day on the job as a "real nurse" not only is exciting, but also extremely stressful! Along with the relief of not having an instructor peering over your shoulder, watching your every move, you may feel a bit of fear at being solely responsible for the care of your patients, and doing—in real life—procedures you may have performed once, or maybe just talked about, during school! Instead of carefully supervised, controlled situations, you are now on your own. To add to the stress, you will probably be working with people you've never met before. Add to that not knowing where the stock meds or IV supplies are kept, or how to order a STAT med—or even where the bathroom is—those first few days on a new job can be pretty hectic.

Whether you are a brand new nurse starting your first job, or an experienced nurse starting your twenty-first job, these hints and tips will make those first days easier.

*Orientation:* Orientation at best consists of several days or weeks of closely monitored patient care, where the new nurse works with another nurse and has the opportunity to ask questions, practice procedures with supervision, obtain help as needed, and find out the secrets of how the facility functions ("Don't call Dr. Jones after 10PM unless his patient is coding; Dr. Webster makes rounds at 6AM."). Unfortunately, orientation sometimes consists of "The charts are over here and the patients are down the hall."

During your interview, ask about the length of orientation and what it includes. After you start your new job, don't be afraid to insist on an extra day of orientation if you don't feel you've obtained necessary basic information, or you feel very unsure of policies and the floor routine. Remember, though, that you will have some unease the first time you work without direct supervision, no matter how experienced you are or long your orientation has been. Take an *active* part in orientation; ask lots of questions, observe any procedures that you can (even if not on your patients), and ask another nurse to critique your techniques which you are uncomfortable with.

*Know your job description:* Job descriptions and responsibilities—even for the same job title—may differ from facility to facility. Along with your written job description, ask your Charge Nurse which tasks you may ask another ancillary staff member (nurses aid, unit secretary) to perform.

If you are a Team Leader, be aware of what your team members can do (IV's, tube feedings, IV medications, and so on). If you are a Team Member, know which tasks your Team Leader can help you with—tracking down lab results, calling doctors, etc. By knowing your job description, you can perform your job much more efficiently.

If your job description should change; for example, you are promoted to night Charge Nurse, don't be afraid to ask for additional orientation.

After Mary Beth had worked the day shift on the pediatrics unit for six months, she requested a transfer to the night shift. As one of the night RN's was on maternity leave, she was asked to be the night

Charge Nurse. Although Mary Beth was comfortable with the routine of the day shift on that floor, she wasn't familiar with the night routine or the responsibilities of a night Charge Nurse. After she expressed her concerns to the Head Nurse, Mary Beth learned the Charge Nurse duties while another experienced Charge Nurse showed her the routine, and answered her questions. After just three nights, Mary Beth was ready to be on her own!

*Dress for success:* During your tour of the area in which you will be working, observe the nurses' dress code. Look to see if the nurses wear dress clothes, uniforms, caps, nursing shoes or aerobic shoes, and/or lab coats.

Elizabeth noticed the nurses and counselors wearing jeans and casual T-shirts on her tour of the children's psych unit she hoped to work on. She accepted the job she was offered, and decided to make a good impression by wearing a skirt and high heels her first day of work. Unfortunately, this backfired when she was asked to join the kids and other nurses and counselors in a game of dodge ball during activity time. If you are unsure of the dress code, ask your supervisor—*before* your first day!

*Beat the bell:* Even veteran nurses will benefit from arriving 15 minutes prior to the start of the shift for the first several days or weeks of a new job. Use this time to locate IV supplies, stock drugs, and other supplies you will be using. Familiarize yourself with the routines of the unit; how the phones work *(before* you disconnect a doctor in the middle of a conversation), which doctors do rounds early or late, how the charts are arranged, unit policies and procedures, etc. New grads can use this time to organize their patient assignment and look up procedures or medications they are unfamiliar with.

The inconvenience of arriving early will be outweighed by how quickly you feel more at ease with the routine of the unit. However, check facility policy regarding "clock in" time. Some facilities and managers do not want you to clock in prior to the time the shift begins, regardless of your intentions. You do not want to be reprimanded for being "on the clock" too early when all you are attempting to do is become familiar with the unit. Keep in mind that "beating the bell" may have to be done on *your* time.

*Get organized:* Many nurses find that a clipboard is a valuable way to keep information together. Some nurses write down minimal information to keep them on track, and other nurses feel more comfortable writing down every detail. Ask other nurses how they organize their notes; use the ideas you like and make your own organization sheet.

After finding out—the hard way!—that even seemingly routine procedures vary from facility to facility, Anne made checklists for tasks that needed to be completed upon admission, dismissal, transfer, and sending a patient to the OR. She taped the checklists to her clipboard, where they were immediately available for reference. After several weeks she was familiar with what needed to be done, but it was reassuring to be able to double check.

*Don't be shy:* Be nice to everyone! Experienced employees, from every department, can give you valuable information. Mike, new to the telemetry unit, was friendly to everyone he encountered. The Unit Secretary soon taught him the secrets of using the telephone and intercom system; Tom, the monitor tech, taught him how to print off a rhythm strip and review any abnormal rhythms by familiarizing him with the monitor equipment; Pat from the pharmacy showed him how to order a STAT medication through the computer; and Stephanie, the housekeeper, showed him where the extra pillows and blankets were. It would have taken Mike weeks to learn these time-saving tips on his own. People responded to Mike's friendliness by gladly sharing their knowledge with him, and thus made his orientation much smoother and quicker.

*Help and you will be helped:* Deb only had two patients to care for during her first week of orientation. When she was caught up with her tasks, she offered to help other nurses who were busy. When they got over their surprise at her willingness to help, they were more than willing to show her how to work the feeding pumps and give her advice on dealing with difficult doctors and getting phone calls returned.

*Judge not . . .* Judge fellow nurses for yourself. When Ashley began her new job in Labor and Delivery, several of the nurses didn't like working with one particular nurse. Ashley decided to judge Whitney for herself. Although Whitney was rather opinionated and had her own way of doing things, Ashley found her to be a very good teacher who gave excellent patient care. Whitney's experience and willingness to teach made those first few weeks a lot easier for Ashley, and although they no longer work in the same hospital, they are still good friends.

*Let's eat!* Bring a sack lunch *and* money the first several days of your new job, at least until you know the routine of the area in which you are working. In some areas there is almost always time for meals, while in others you may have to eat on the run and not have time to go to the cafeteria.    Whether you are new to the profession, or just new to the facility, remember that it takes several months to become really comfortable in a new job. By accepting this, you won't feel so stressed out about *feeling* stressed out about your new job. Remember to do nice things for *yourself* during this time; leave your job at work, relax by going for a walk or taking a warm bath, or doing something else *you* enjoy. One day, you'll walk into work and discover you are comfortable after all!

# Oops! It's Not Your Perfect Job . . .

*". . . use every job situation to grow and develop personally and professionally."* Jean Beyer, R.N.

*Unit dynamics:* One of the most interesting aspects of each new job is the unique way each particular area functions and relates interpersonally among staff members, managers, and department heads. Often, this alone can make or break your happiness with a particular job. While it is impossible to fully assess this information in the brief amount of time during an interview and in touring an area, do keep your antenna up and do not let obvious cues and clues pass without detection simply because the job fits, for example, your scheduling needs.

For instance, if a potential manager interviewing you asks several pointed questions related to how you would handle aggressive and difficult staff members who are currently employed by the facility, instead of planning an impressive answer, you should be wondering why the manager herself hasn't dealt with these employees! This is a definite red flag—take heed!

Okay, so you didn't see that red flag . . . The job was offered and you asked for the necessary time to think it over (a minimum of 24-48 hours is recommended). During this time you mulled over all the information and it *did* seem like the Perfect Job—it fit all of your criteria—so why did you feel so unsettled about accepting it? You may have decided to formulate some questions to ask the manager, about any concerns related to the job, prior to accepting the job. This was appropriate; remember, there was a *reason* for your sense of discomfort.

During your time to "think it over," remember to "feel it over," and trust your own instincts. Chances are, your own gut feeling will turn out to be correct! There is little else more disheartening than finding out your Perfect Job is in an unhappy and unhealthy unit that takes the "fun" right out of "dysfunctional"!

*Cutting your losses:* So perhaps you are in a job which is not right for you—you forgot to "feel it over," or perhaps you were just plain fooled! The result is the same— you are unhappy! You have not met your needs for professionalism and self-fulfillment. Don't brow-beat yourself or disregard all the strategies you have learned. Recognize what didn't work, address it, and move on and resolve not to repeat mistakes. You may simply need to spend more time perfecting your evaluation of the unit dynamics area. Regardless of the reason, should you find yourself in an area that is intolerable to you because it goes against your nursing ethics (such as patient safety violations), or jeopardizes your personal safety, you *must* take action! Express your concerns in a respectful manner, to the appropriate person.

Currently legislation is being proposed (HR3355, or the Patient Safety Act), which would give nurses avenues of recourse for facilities which blatantly disregard patient safety issues. Until this legislation is in place, either ask for a transfer to another area within the facility, or quietly begin your job search anew. Never stay in an area which is unhappy and unhealthy for you professionally, or in which your personal safety is at risk. Work as diligently and quickly as possible to locate another area or facility for employment. Don't be discouraged by this minor setback! Fortunately, the odds are against your being employed in another dysfunctional unit, especially now that your "radar" is heightened and you will be more aware of the impact unit dynamics plays in your successful employment. You will certainly be more attentive in your observations during subsequent interviews and tours!

A job which jeopardizes your licensure by promoting unsafe nursing care, or degrades your own personal and sacred vow as the patient advocate, is never worth your sacrifices to keep! Cut your losses—save your license, your health, your heartache and your pride and walk away; but, do it by *your* choice, with your dignity intact, and without burning any bridges.

> *"When I do change jobs, I like it to be in a totally different area. I needed to see patients go home everyday. I don't dread going to work every morning now."* Terry Lasseter, R.N.

*Burning bridges:* Do give notice (the customary two-week notice is sufficient) and exit as soon as possible.

No matter how tempting it may be to walk out or tell everyone what you *really* think of them during your last days, resist this temptation! You may seek employment at that facility in the future, or your current supervisor or co-workers may, at some time, work in another facility in which you are employed. Your mother *was* right—no matter how much you hate to hear it (and *really* want to get it off your chest), "if you can't say anything nice, don't say anything at all." There are much more constructive things on which you should be concentrating—like lobbying for HR3355 or focusing on your new job search!

# One Final Note

All of this information was compiled to help you choose your path wisely. We are, after all, nurses! We want not only to take care of you, but to teach you to take care of yourselves! Welcome to nursing!

# Appendix

# Nursing Opportunities Requiring Additional Education

Even with all of the current issues related to health reform, most health-care experts are predicting continuing strong opportunities for nursing employment, particularly in the areas of Home Health, Out-Patient Services, and middle management.

There are a variety of educational paths you may take to become a nurse. Below is a listing of the approximate time commitment necessary for each "degree" of licensed nursing.

*Education Requirements:*

LPN Licensed Practical Nurse 1-1½ years

Degrees providing Registered Nurse licensure:

| | |
|---|---|
| ADN Associate Degree in Nursing | 2 years |
| Diploma (program usually hospital based) | 3 years |
| BSN Bachelor of Science in Nursing | 4 years |
| MSN Masters of Science in Nursing | 6 years |
| PhD Doctorate of Nursing (a Doctor Nurse!) | 8 years |

The time requirements listed here are general requirements; some programs may require more or less time. Of course, if you choose to attend school part-time, it will take longer, and if you choose to take a heavy class load, it may take a shorter period of time.

A BSN is preferred for many management jobs, and advanced degrees (MSN, PhD) open up advanced teaching, research, and "theory" jobs.

*Certification:* As well as the above mentioned degrees, there are even more numerous certifications for nurses. Certification gives you "added value" by showing a level of experience and expertise in the area of certification. To become certified, a nurse must meet certain requirements of education and experience, and pass a certifying examination. The exam questions are provided by certified nurses, and include questions regarding theory and practice in the specific certification area. Effective with the 1998 certification tests, a BSN, or even higher, will be required for certification in even general areas. Certification prior to 1998 will remain available to nurses without a BSN, as long as the certification is renewed every five years.

For more (free!) information regarding requirements and test schedules, contact the American Nurses Credentialing Center at 1-800-284-CERT.

*Advanced Practice Opportunities:* Many of you will decide to continue on in nursing in what is known as Advanced Practice Nursing. This includes Nurse Anesthetists, Nurse Practitioners, Clinical Nurse Specialists, and Nurse Midwives. All require additional education and training beyond an ADN or BSN. Requirements are as follows:

*Nurse Anesthetist:* Most schools of anesthesia require applicants to have a BSN, and two additional years of study are required to be a Certified Registered Nurse Anesthetist (CRNA). The majority of anesthetists are employed in hospitals. CRNA's are the third largest group of Advanced Practice Nurses.

*Nurse Practitioner:* Nurse Practitioners must have an MSN. Sub-specialties include Family, School, Pediatric, Geriatric, and Adult Care Nurse Practitioners. 58% of Nurse Practitioners are certified. This is the second largest group of Advanced Practice Nurses.

*Clinical Specialist:* This area also requires an MSN, and sub-specialties include Med/Surg, Gerontological, Community Health, Home Health, Adult Psychiatric and Mental Health, and Child and Adolescent Psychiatric and Mental Health Nursing. The Clinical Specialist is usually employed by a hospital, and teaches staff and patients. This is the largest group of Advanced Practice Nurses.

*Nurse Midwife:* Nurse Midwives are the smallest group of Advanced Practice Nurses. Requirements include a basic nursing education and nine months (no pun intended!) of additional experience and education. Nurse Midwives may be independently employed or employed by birthing centers or hospitals. About 2/3 are certified.

*Professional Organizations:* The American Nurses Credentialing Center (ANCC) was established in 1973 by the American Nurses Association (ANA). The ANA is nurses' professional organization which lobbies for Health Reform legislation impacting nursing, as well as the health care consumer. Let your voice be heard! Join the ANA and attend and participate in any ANA activity. For more information regarding the ANA call(202) 651-7180 or contact your state nurses association.

Other professional organizations also offer their own peer review exams for the purpose of acknowledging individuals who meet specialized standards of care in a certain area.

*Salaries:* One additional aspect to consider is salaries. It is interesting to note that salaries are not always commensurate with educational levels. Currently, CRNA's hold the distinction of being the highest paid within the nursing profession, with a salary range from $28-30 per hour. Supervisors earn from $22-30 per hour, Nurse practitioners $21-30 per hour, and Head Nurses $21-29 per hour. These are the four highest paid nursing positions, as recorded by the U.S. Department of Labor, Bureau of Labor Statistics in the 1991 study.

So you see, the sky is the limit! And in fact, as a flight nurse, you can even nurse *in* the sky! Choose your path and get going—to Your Perfect Job in Nursing.

# Acronym Index

| | |
|---|---|
| ACLS | Advanced Cardiac Life Support |
| ADL's | Activities of Daily Living |
| ADN | Associate Degree in Nursing |
| ADON | Assistant Director of Nursing |
| ANA | American Nurses Association |
| ANCC | American Nurses Credentialing Center |
| BSN | Bachelor of Science in Nursing |
| BTLS | Basic Trauma Life Support |
| CC | Critical Care |
| CCRN | Critical Care Registered Nurse |
| CCU | Cardiac Care Unit |
| CNA | Certified Nursing Assistant |
| CPR | Cardio Pulmonary Resuscitation |
| CRNA | Certified Registered Nurse Anesthetist |
| CSM | Care Staff Member |
| CVP | Central Venous Pressure |
| DON | Director of Nursing |
| EKG | Electrocardiogram |
| EMT | Emergency Medical Technician |
| ER | Emergency Room |

| | |
|---|---|
| FHR | Fetal Heart Rate |
| HR | Heart Rate |
| ICU | Intensive Care Unit |
| IV | Intravenous |
| JCAHO | Joint Commission on the Accreditation of Hospitals Organization |
| L & D | Labor and Delivery |
| LPN | Licensed Practical Nurse |
| LTC | Long-term Care |
| MDS | Minimum Data Set |
| MI | Myocardial Infarction |
| MSN | Master of Science in Nursing |
| NG | Naso-gastric |
| NICU | Neonatal Intensive Care Unit |
| OB | Obstetrics |
| OPS | Out-patient Services |
| OR | Operating Room |
| PACU | Post-anesthesia Care Unit |
| PALS | Pediatric Advanced Life Support |
| PCA | Patient Controlled Anesthesia |
| PhD | Doctorate in Nursing |
| PICC | Peripherally Inserted Central Catheter |

| | |
|---|---|
| PICU | Pediatric Intensive Care Unit *or* Post-Intensive Care Unit |
| PTO | Paid Time Off |
| QA | Quality Assurance |
| RN | Registered Nurse |
| RR | Recovery Room |
| TPN | Total Parenteral Nutrition |
| UA | Urinalysis |
| WIC | Women, Infants, Children |

# Can I Write It Off?
# Tax Issues in Nursing

Preparing, printing, and mailing your resume, career counseling, gas and car upkeep, long-distance phone calls to prospective employers, newspapers and nursing magazines purchased to search for job opportunities—job-hunting can be expensive!

You will be happy to learn that all of the above job- hunting expenses are tax-deductible!

Some other job-related expenses are also deductible:

* uniforms, if required by your employer

* cost of medical exam, if required to get, or keep, a job

* professional organization dues

* workshops you attend to obtain required CEU's, or workshops which maintain or improve the skills of your *present* job

These job-related expenses may amount to a large sum of money over the course of a year! Save your receipts and talk with your accountant regarding record-keeping or with any questions you may have.

# Glossary

Arterial blood draw—blood drawn from an artery to determine oxygen content

Activities of Daily Living (ADL's)—eating, dressing, toileting, bathing, etc.

Added Value—all additional skills, education, training and experiences which increase a nurse's potential value to employers

Advanced Cardiac Life Support (ACLS)—life support including the use of drugs, intubation, defibrillation, as well as basic CPR

Amniocentesis—removal of amniotic fluid through a needle inserted abdominally through the uterus; the fluid is analyzed to determine fetal maturity and detect certain disorders

Apnea monitor—machine that monitors a patient's respirations and oxygen level, and alarms if either go above or below pre-set limits

Benefits—services or additional pay offered to employees free or at a reduced rate

Bladder tap—collection of a urine specimen by a needle inserted into the bladder through the abdomen; urine analyzed for diagnostic purposes

Blood draw—obtaining a blood sample for diagnostic purposes

Career ladder—advancement in the nursing structure of a health-care facility

Care Staff Member (CSM)—CNA with additional training allowing him/her to administer certain medications

Central line—a transduced IV inserted into a large blood vessel, to deliver medications, obtain blood specimens, or obtain diagnostic pressure readings

Central Venous Pressure (CVP)—measurement obtained through a central line, which indicates the effectiveness of the heart

Certification—examinations which provide recognition by peers, of professional achievement of theory and application in given nursing areas

Certified Nursing Assistant (CNA)—person trained to obtain vital signs and provide assistance with ADL's

Cervix—opening of the uterus

Chemotherapy—medications, which may be very toxic, usually given for the treatment of cancer

Chest tube—Tube inserted into the chest wall to remove blood and/or air

Circumcision—surgical removal of the foreskin of the penis; usually done within 24 hours of birth

Code—when a patient goes into cardiac and/or respiratory arrest, a "code" is called, paging doctors and specially trained nurses to that patient's room

Contraction—alternate tightening and relaxing of the uterine muscles during labor, causing the cervix to efface and dilate

Contraction Stress Test—assessing the fetus' reaction to contractions by monitoring heart rate and movement

Credit Union—a financial organization whose members may save money, and receive loans at a low interest rate

Cross-train—nurse who is trained to work in different areas of the health care facility; for example, Labor and Delivery and the Nursery, or ICU and ER

Defibrillator—machine used to re-start a patients heart or convert an unstable rhythm using electrical shock(s)

Differential—an increase in the basic amount of pay for working weekend, holiday, evening, or night hours; may be minimal or quite substantial

Dilation—progressive opening of the cervix during labor; full dilation is 10 cm.

Disability/Dismemberment insurance—money paid to an employee if s/he is disabled or loses a limb while at work

Effacement—thinning and shortening of the cervix before and during labor; measured as a percentage, with 100% being fully effaced

Electrocardiogram (EKG)—electrical tracing of the heart's activity; used for diagnostic purposes

Emergency Medical Technician (EMT)—lay-person who, through training, is certified to provide basic pre-hospital care

Episiotomy—incision in the perineum done immediately before birth, to facilitate the birth of the baby

Family Planning Clinic—clinic which offers education about birth control and contraceptives; charges depend on persons income

Fetal Heart Rate (FHR)—number of times the fetal heart beats per minute; normal range is 120-160 beats per minute

Float/floating—working on a floor or in an area other than the one on which the nurse is regularly assigned to work

Fundus—upper portion of the uterus; fundal massage is done through the abdomen to encourage the fundus to clamp down and prevent hemorrhage after the delivery of the baby

Geriatric—elderly

Groshong—a type of peripherally Inserted Central Catheter

Gynecology—study of female diseases and problems, especially concerning the reproductive organs and breasts

Heimlich Maneuver—procedure to dislodge an object from the airway of a victim who is choking

Hemodialysis (acute and chronic)—clearing waste products from the blood when the kidneys are ineffective or non-functional

Hospice—supportive care provided to patients with a terminal illness and less than six months to live

Housing Allowance—money given to an employee to rent or buy an apartment or house

Immunization Clinic—clinic providing immunizations at reduced cost or free of charge

Infus-a-ports—implanted port attached to a catheter terminating in the superior vena cava; used for long-term IV access

Inservice—education for nurses, CSM's, CNA's; required by state and federal regulations and usually provided by the facility in which the nurse, CSM, CNA is employed

Interpersonal skills—communication skills used in getting along with others

Leadership skills—actions that assist members of a group to achieve certain goals

Lochia—vaginal discharge of the mother after the birth of a baby; excess may indicate hemorrhage; lasts for several weeks after the baby's birth

Management skills—those actions necessary to oversee all aspects of meeting a group's goals

Meals on Wheels—program in which meals are delivered to people who are unable to leave their homes and/or find cooking very difficult

Mission Statement—a facility's statement of purpose and philosophy

Nasogastric (NG)—tube inserted orally or nasally to provide food or nutrition, or remove the contents of the stomach

Neonatal Intensive Care Unit (NICU)—unit in which critically ill premature babies or newborns are cared for

Neurology—care of patients with problems or diseases related to the nervous system

Non-stress Test—test in which fetal health is evaluated by monitoring FHR and movement

On-call—nurse must be available to return to the health-care facility if needed during "on-call" hours

Oncology—care of patients whose primary diagnosis is cancer

Orientation—the process of familiarizing new employees to the facility's policies and procedures, mission statement, benefits, physical layout, etc.

Orthopedics—care of patients with problems of bones, muscles, ligaments, etc.

Oximeter—non-invasive device which determines the amount of oxygen in the blood

Pacemaker—device implanted under the skin in the chest area, which electrically paces the heart

Paid Time Off—traditionally time off with pay, encompasses "sick", "vacation," "Holiday Pay," etc., and used at the employee's discretion within facility guidelines

Patient Controlled Anesthesia (PCA)—device in which the patient is able to control the amount of pain medication s/he receives through an IV

Pediatric—patients up to the age of 18 years

Pediatric Advanced Life Support (PALS)—ACLS when performed on a pediatric patient

Pension Plan—a benefit which is a regular, non-wage payment to an employee, based on criteria such as retirement, disability, etc.

Peri-care—cleansing of the perineal area in patients who are unable to do this themselves

Peripheral—pertaining to a vessel in the arm or hand

Peripherally Inserted Central Catheter—a type of IV catheter inserted peripherally into the superior vena cava; used for long-term IV access for medication, blood administration, TPN, etc.

Pulmonary Function Test—tests which determine the function of a patient's lungs

Recruitment Bonus—money an employee may receive when hired to work at a health-care facility, or money an employee may receive when recruiting another employee to work at that facility

Rejection—a term related to transplantation; when the body's immune system recognizes the new organ as "foreign" and fights the new organ with a normal immune defense response

Relocation Assistance—money a new employee may receive to help defray costs of moving

Reverse Isolation—when the caregiver is considered to be contaminated and is cloaked in isolation protective gear to protect the patient's weakened immune system

Right and Left Atrial Pressure Lines—transduced indwelling catheter lines which are inserted during open-heart surgery to measure heart function immediately after surgery

Scrubs—work clothes that may be provided and/or laundered by the hospital or the employee; usually worn in specialized areas; critical care, ER, surgery, etc.

Self-catheterization—the procedure of draining the bladder, performed by the patient requiring frequent and long-term catheterization

Shift Differential—money an employee receives above basic pay for working evening, night, or weekend shifts

Spinal Tap—procedure in which spinal fluid is collected through a needle inserted into the lower portion of the spinal canal; fluid is analyzed for diagnostic purposes

Swan-Ganz—central venous lines which measure right sided heart pressure, and lung pressures

T-Pieces—a "T" shaped connector which fits standard ventilator tubing

Target Area(s)—those areas in which a nurses wishes to concentrate his or her job search

Technical Skills—mechanical, "hands on" skills needed to perform a specific job

Telemetry—monitoring of a patient's heart rate and rhythm through electrodes attached to the patients chest and a box which transmits information to a central location

Total Parenteral Nutrition—meeting a patient's nutritional needs through his or her IV

Triage—determining which patients' conditions require treatment most urgently

Universal Precautions—use of gloves, gown, and/or mask to avoid contact with the blood or body fluids of any patient

Urinalysis—analyzing urine for diagnostic purposes

Vaginal Shave—removing, by shaving, the hair around the vaginal area

Ventilator—machine which "breathes" for a patient who is unable to

Well-child Clinic—clinic in which healthy children can be evaluated and assessed

Women, Infants, Children—program in which low-income families can receive food

**Yes!** Send me *How to Find Your Perfect Job in Nursing!*

Name _____

Address _____

City _____

State _____ Zip _____

Phone ( _____ ) _____

Please send me _____ copies of *How to Find Your Perfect Job in Nursing,* at $25 each. (NE residents add $1.25 for state tax plus city tax where applicable)

**Shipping & Handling:** $3 for one book; $2 for each additional book (free shipping and handling for orders of 20 books or more to the same address.)

I have enclosed $ _____ .

Please make checks out to:

**SHELMAR PUBLICATIONS.**

For Visa or MasterCard orders, call (402) 993-9903.

Your book will arrive in approximately 4-6 weeks.

30 day money-back guarantee if you are not completely satisfied with *How to Find Your Perfect Job in Nursing.*

**Comments or Suggestions:**